Behavioral Change in Cerebrovascular Disease

Behavioral Change in Cerebrovascular Disease

Edited by ARTHUR L. BENTON, Ph.D.

University of Iowa, Iowa City

BY 22 AUTHORS

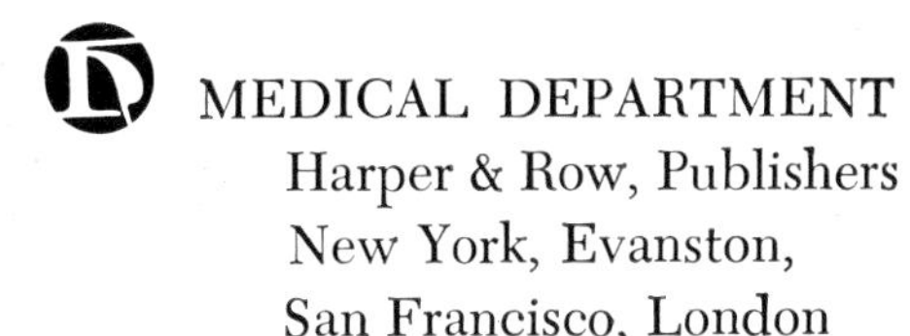

MEDICAL DEPARTMENT
Harper & Row, Publishers
New York, Evanston,
San Francisco, London

 Printed in the United States of America. For information address Medical Department, Harper & Row, Publishers, Inc., 49 East 33rd Street, New York, N.Y. 10016.

FIRST EDITION

STANDARD BOOK NUMBER: 06-140424-1
LIBRARY OF CONGRESS CATALOG CARD NUMBER: 73-133136

CONTENTS

LIST OF WORKSHOP PARTICIPANTS

JEAN N. ANGELO, M.D. Laboratory of Neuropathology, Boston Veterans Administration Hospital, Boston, Massachusetts

A. B. BAKER, M.D. Professor of Neurology and Head, Division of Neurology, University of Minnesota Medical School, Minneapolis

RAYMOND B. BAUER, M.D. Professor of Neurology, Wayne State University School of Medicine, Detroit, Michigan

D. FRANK BENSON, M.D. Clinical Director, Aphasia Research Center, and Associate Professor of Neurology, Boston University School of Medicine, Boston, Massachusetts

ARTHUR L. BENTON, Ph.D. Professor of Psychology and Neurology, University of Iowa, Iowa City

FREDERIC L. DARLEY, Ph.D. Chief, Section of Speech Pathology, Department of Neurology, Mayo Clinic, Rochester, Minnesota

LEONARD DILLER, Ph.D. Chief, Behavioral Science Division, Institute of Rehabilitation Medicine, and Associate Professor of Rehabilitation Medicine, New York University School of Medicine, New York

NORMAN GESCHWIND, M.D. James Jackson Putnam Professor of Neurology, Harvard Medical School, and Director, Neurological Unit, Boston City Hospital, Boston, Massachusetts

MURRAY GOLDSTEIN, D.O., M.P.H. Associate Director for Extramural Programs, National Institute for Neurological Diseases and Stroke, Bethesda, Maryland

HAROLD GOODGLASS, Ph.D. Director, Psychology Research, Boston Veterans Administration Hospital, Boston, Massachusetts

GLENN GULLICKSON, JR., M.D. Professor of Physical Medicine and Rehabilitation, University of Minnesota Medical School, Minneapolis

SIMON HORENSTEIN, M.D. Professor and Chief, Section of Neurology, St. Louis University School of Medicine, St. Louis, Missouri

ROBERT J. JOYNT, M.D. Professor of Neurology, University of Rochester

School of Medicine and Dentistry, and Neurologist-in-Chief, Strong Memorial Hospital, Rochester, New York

FLETCHER H. MCDOWELL, M.D. Associate Professor of Neurology, Cornell University Medical College, New York, New York

MANFRED J. MEIER, Ph.D. Professor, Departments of Psychology and Neurosurgery, University of Minnesota, Minneapolis

CLARK H. MILLIKAN, M.D. Senior Neurologist, Mayo Clinic, and Professor of Neurology, Mayo Graduate School of Medicine (University of Minnesota), Rochester, Minnesota

JOHN MOOSSY, M.D. Professor of Neuropathology, The Bowman Gray School of Medicine of Wake Forest University, Winston-Salem, North Carolina

RALPH M. REITAN, Ph.D. Professor of Psychology and Neurological Surgery, University of Washington, Seattle

A. L. SAHS, M.D. Professor and Head, Department of Neurology, University of Iowa College of Medicine, Iowa City

RICHARD SATRAN, M.D. Associate Professor of Neurology, University of Rochester School of Medicine and Dentistry, Rochester, New York

MALVINA SCHWEIZER, Ph.D. Office of Director, National Heart Institute, Bethesda, Maryland

JOSE M. SEGARRA, M.D. Chief of Neuropathology, Boston Veterans Administration Hospital, Boston, Massachusetts

DONALD P. SHANKWEILER, Ph.D. Associate Professor of Psychology, University of Connecticut School of Medicine, and Research Associate, Haskins Laboratories, New Haven, Connecticut

OTFRIED SPREEN, Ph.D. Professor of Psychology, University of Victoria, British Columbia, Canada

PETER H. STERN, M.D. Assistant Clinical Professor in Medicine (Rehabilitation), Cornell University Medical College, and Physician-in-Chief, Physical Medicine, Burke Rehabilitation Center, White Plains, New York

MAURICE W. VAN ALLEN, M.D. Professor of Neurology and Director, Neurosensory Center, University of Iowa College of Medicine, Iowa City

PREFACE

This book contains the edited proceedings of a workshop on behavioral change in cerebrovascular disease which was held in Swampscott, Massachusetts, in September 1968. The workshop was sponsored by the Joint Council Subcommittee on Cerebrovascular Diseases of the National Institute of Neurological Diseases and Stroke, and the National Heart Institute. This volume has three aims: to provide a critical assessment of our present understanding of the determinants and nature of the behavioral changes associated with cerebrovascular disease; to identify problems that remain unresolved and require further investigation; and to consider research strategies that will help solve these problems.

The distinguished contributors to this collective work have focused their attention not only on questions of immediate interest to the clinician, but also on the theoretical issues that provide a rational basis for the prediction, prevention, and management of the behavioral deficits of patients with cerebrovascular disease.

The behavioral disabilities that occur as a consequence of cerebrovascular disease take a variety of forms: general mental impairment ("dementia"); specific cognitive, perceptual, or psychomotor deficits indicative of a focal lesion; emotional changes and personality disorders; and disturbances of speech and language. This last group of disabilities is of particular importance. As Geschwind points out in Presentation 4, aphasic disorder frequently is the only residual disability shown by the patient who has suffered from stroke, or else the sole handicap that prevents him from making a satisfactory social and economic adjustment.

Among the questions still unanswered concerning these disabilities are the precise nature of the anatomical and physiological mechanisms involved in the production of behavioral change; problems of localization that are of both theoretical and practical diagnostic import; the effectiveness of rehabilitation procedures; the usefulness of psychological test procedures in detecting, predicting, and monitoring behavioral change; and the significance of the personality alterations manifested by some stroke patients. Since the authors are themselves active researchers in the field, their contributions are based on a first-hand appreciation of the key problems involved.

I am deeply indebted to Drs. Norman Geschwind, Robert J. Joynt, and John Moossy, who shared responsibility for planning the program, and to Dr. Murray Goldstein and Dr. Jerome G. Green for their advice and encouragement during the course of the project. I am grateful to Marilyn Lang whose aid in reviewing and processing the manuscript significantly lightened my task as editor.

Because of its medical, social, and economic importance, the steadily increasing incidence of cerebrovascular disease makes this effort a particularly timely one. It is our hope that it will fill the need for which it is intended.

Iowa City, Iowa

ARTHUR L. BENTON

SECTION I

Anatomical Determinants of Behavioral Change

PRESENTATION 1

Jose M. Segarra
Jean N. Angelo

The scope and purpose of this presentation are to discuss the role of the pathologist in the study of abnormal behavior, or in other words, to define the types and extent of pathological changes underlying alterations in behavior. In a sense, one could say that any stroke, any lesion of the brain due to cerebrovascular disease, leads to behavioral changes in the person so affected. Since we cannot review here the entire contribution of neuropathology to the understanding of behavior, we have decided to illustrate this contribution by reporting in detail the anatomical basis of a particular behavioral state, namely, akinetic mutism.

METHODOLOGY

The study of cerebrovascular disease is particularly suitable for investigation of the correlation between function and structure in the nervous system of man. In fact, the "golden age" of neurological analysis stemmed from careful study of vascular lesions for the most part, and indeed laid down the foundation upon which clinical neurology is based. The pathology of human behavior can be examined by the same kind of study. Some truisms can be expressed at the outset: (1) there is no substitute for long patience and the slow accumulation of suitable cases; (2) the contribution of the pathologist will not be significant unless there has been careful study in life; (3) the process of mapping out the extent of the lesions involves the use of serial sections of celloidin-embedded material. Preferably the whole brain should be processed, following the method used at the Warren Museum of Harvard Medical School. We are indebted to Dr. Yakovlev for his kindness in making this technique available to us. Study of material prepared in this way is essential for two reasons: (1) it is the only reliable method for the study of white matter, for, unlike the case with gray matter, gross inspection alone can easily overlook the presence of abnormally modified white tissue, and staining is required; (2) secondary degenerations, organization gliosis, and minute vascular changes may be significant in a particular case.

THE VASCULAR BASIS OF AKINETIC MUTISM

Akinetic mutism has been linked to upper brain-stem lesions since 1941, when the first report by Cairns and his coworkers was published. Most of the studies of human cases, however, have suffered from the fact that lesions held responsible have been either too large or too numerous. The present report deals with cases of akinetic mutism due to single, strikingly small, and well-delimited lesions. The important behavioral repercussions of such discrete lesions represent a true experiment of nature which may throw some light on our understanding of the anatomical substrate of consciousness. Moreover, the relation of such a lesion to an identifiable vascular territory constitutes a recognizable clinical entity or vascular syndrome.

A striking feature of many published reports is the uniformity (or at least the superficial resemblance) of the clinical picture in spite of great diversity of lesions. Cravioto, Silberman, and Feigen (1960) have remarked on this: Diffuse lesions in their case of carbon monoxide poisoning were responsible for an altered state of consciousness essentially similar to that produced by basilar artery occlusion with infarction of the pons. We have observed a similar state in elderly patients who have no obvious lesions but suffer from general debility as a result of infection, dehydration, anemia, or other medical disorder; in these patients the state of consciousness returned to normal when the underlying disease was corrected.

It seems reasonable to assume, therefore, that akinetic mutism is a term which has been used to describe different processes of widely differing mechanism. We will attempt to clarify the concept and to bring out the differential clinical features associated with different localizations.

DEFINITION OF AKINETIC MUTISM

Akinetic mutism is defined as a state of unresponsiveness to the environment with extreme reluctance to perform even elementary motor activities. The patient lies quietly in bed, immobile, sometimes sleepy but often open-eyed and seemingly alert. On occasion his gaze may follow the examiner, but he will not react to the examiner's presence or to any stimuli except painful ones. He has no real awareness of the events around him. This state shows gradations in severity. Powerful stimuli may elicit movements, and even speech, but the patient readily sinks back into a state variously described as indifference, lacking in social awareness, lacking in will, lethargy, or somnolence. Yet, for all this detachment from the world around, the expression of the patient's eyes often gives the observer a subjective impression of awareness and of stubborn refusal to cooperate.

We may classify such patients in two broad categories: pseudoakinetic mutes and true akinetic mutes. The following is a discussion of both.

PSEUDOAKINETIC MUTE STATES

The "Sentient Mummy" Syndrome. A pseudoakinetic mute state may accompany basilar artery occlusion with pontine infarction. This is actually a state of paralysis resulting from interruption of descending motor pathways to the spinal cord as well as to lower cranial nerve nuclei; only the ocular movements remain, and communication by blinking is possible. An excellent account of such cases has been given by Kemper and Romanul (1967). The state has been termed "the locked-in syndrome" by Plum and Posner (1966). Kemper and Romanul wisely described it as "resembling akinetic mutism" and urged that the distinction between paralysis and akinesia be kept in mind. On clinical, anatomical, and physiological grounds this state has little relation to our subject. To use the terms akinesia and mutism for what is in fact merely paralysis from bilateral upper motor neuron disease is to introduce conceptual confusion. This paralytic state is discussed in the literature under the term "akinetic mutism," even though it is evident from the descriptions that the patients are conscious and can carry on two-way communication with the world, even of a complex nature, by codified blinking of the eyes. Most of the cases of Cravioto, Silberman, and Feigin (1960), as well as Case 1 of Fang and Palmer (1956), are of this type.

Mutism of Extrapyramidal Origin. Almost all the known diseases of the basal ganglia end in a state of extreme hypokinesia, rigidity, and mutism. In the realm of cerebrovascular disease, symmetrical destruction of putamen, caudate, and/or globus pallidus has been observed repeatedly as a cause of such states. Denny-Brown (1962a) quotes Marinesco and Draganesco's description of a boy with necrosis of the putamen and caudate following seizure who would lie in an unresponsive state, mute and without purposeful movements. Another report describes a child who would not speak or respond to commands, but whose eyes would follow the movements of another person. Pallidal necrosis not associated with other lesions has been reported by Denny-Brown to lead to an akinetic state. All such cases are the result of a mixture of rigidity and pseudobulbar symptomatology. Relatively pure pallidal lesions can be found in carbon monoxide poisoning. Chemopallidectomy for Parkinson's disease occasionally results in mutism after the remaining globus pallidus is destroyed during a second operation. These and similar cases bear a superficial resemblance to akinetic mutism *sensu strictu*. The mixture of rigidity, dysphagia, dyslalia, tongue paralysis, bilateral extensor plantar reflexes, and occasional outbursts of pseudobulbar affect makes the distinction possible on clinical grounds alone.

The "Apallic State" of Kretschmer. Another state which closely resembles akinetic mutism ensues from almost complete destruction of the pallium, or mantle zone, of the hemispheric convexity. Earlier we suggested the term "pallio-prive state" for such a condition, but in the interest of euphony decided to keep Kretschmer's original denomination. The apallic state may result from anoxia, carbon monoxide poisoning, degenerative disease such as the Jakob-Creutzfeldt syndrome, meningovascular syphilis (French, 1952, Case 5), chronic viral encephalitis, or closed-head trauma. Clinically the patient appears mute and immobile, with wide-open eyes which may follow the observer for a short period of time, but more often than not roam at random.

It seems reasonable to assume that a mechanism different from that operating in patients with mesencephalic lesions, as in the cases reported below, is responsible for this state, for the akinesia and unresponsiveness are the result of direct injury to secondary and associative sensorimotor areas with relative preservation of the archipallium and, perhaps, primary motor areas. There is no defect in the will, no lethargy, no lack of social awareness as patients with frontal or mesencephalic lesions, but the necessary substrate for felling, movement, or thought is absent. Since only the most elementary reactions are elicitable, the patient is akinetic and mute. These patients often show marked alterations in muscle tone and posture which may help in differentiating them from patients with true akinetic mutism. The patients discussed by Jellinger, Gerstenbrand, and Pateisky (1963) belong in the apallic group.

TRUE AKINETIC MUTE STATES

The states described below constitute true akinetic mutism, or akinetic mutism *sensu strictu*, since in these patients akinesia and mutism appear without paralysis or gross motor and sensory alterations and with an intact neopallium.

Akinetic Mutism of Cingulate Origin. This term designates the akinetic states secondary to lesions in the medial surfaces of one or both frontal lobes.

Occlusion of the anterior cerebral arteries followed by infarction or hemorrhage may lead to coma or to a state similar to akinetic mutism. The participation of the anterior cingulate region (area 24) seems to be the most important factor in the production of the syndrome.

There are, however, significant variations in the extent of apathy and unresponsiveness of patients with medial frontal lesions. Faris (1967) described a young girl with hemorrhagic destruction of the cingulate cortex in whom severe withdrawal alternated with intermittent bouts of agitation and screaming. This intermittent agitation with aimless aggressivity is perhaps the most distinctive feature of frontal lobe akinesia. Another feature is the patient's ability occasionally to give short monosyllabic but intelligent answers.

Neighborhood signs are, of course, most helpful, and evidence of focal motor disabilities (seizures, monoplegia, hemiplegia, etc.) strongly suggest frontal lobe disease rather than brain-stem lesions. Nielsen and Jacobs (1951) and Amyes and Nielsen (1955) described similar cases. Barris and Schuman (1953) reported another observation of the same type. It is evident from their description that the main symptom is apathy which progresses to stupor and coma. Bilateral extensor plantar reflexes are a common feature.

One pertinent comment, which Barris and Schuman made in their paper, is the apparent paradox between the fulminating symptomatology of cingulate destruction by vascular disease and the lack of such effects after surgical excisions, e.g., for psychiatric indications. The reason is not clear, but may have something to do with the extent and the timing of lesional development. In essence, therefore, the akinetic state of frontal lesion origin is a "vigilant" one and contrasts with the "somnolent" akinetic state of subthalamic lesions (Yakovlev, 1968).

Akinetic Mutism of Mesencephalic Origin. Lesions responsible for akinetic mutism have been localized within the broad limits of the thalamomesencephalic junction, but the precise site of the responsible lesion has eluded most students of this subject, since the majority of published cases are the result of tumor, encephalitis, trauma, or extensive infarction.

We intend to show in this report that akinetic mutism may be the result of strikingly minute, thin, elongated infarcts lying across the caudal-most portion of the third ventricle just above the mesencephalic tegmentum and spreading butterfly-fashion at the border between the inferior thalamus and the subthalamic area. The whole lesion is a slit not more than 2 mm. thick and 6 mm. wide.

Two cases with the clinical picture of akinetic mutism have been studied in our laboratory using serial sections of celloidin-embedded material from the thalamomesencephalic junction. Both cases are almost identical in the extent, topography, and nature of the lesions. The formations destroyed include: (1) the medial third of the centrum medianum, (2) the lower third of the midline thalamic nuclei, (3) the nucleus parafascicularis and the reticular nucleus of the lamina medullaris interna, (4) the periventricular gray matter in the floor of the third ventricle, and (5) the mesencephalic midline reticular nuclei at the caudal tip of the brain stem.

DISCUSSION OF PREVIOUSLY REPORTED CASES

A review of the literature on akinetic mutism has been presented by Klee (1961) and need not be repeated here. Most of the cases have been characterized by widespread and rather massive pathology not suitable to precise localization. Cairns' (1941) original observation dealt with a tumor situated in the *anterior* portion of the third ventricle. Since then, a variety of lesions have been associated with this condition, e.g., epidermoid cysts, metastatic tumors, angiomas, trauma, Wernicke's disease, and encephalitis.

Perusal of this material shows clearly that patients with vascular disease, especially ischemic infarction, are the most appropriate subjects in which to study this condition. Even so, most of the reported observations pertain to rather massive vascular lesions of the brain stem which may or may not be related to akinetic mutism, as discussed above. However, a limited number of cases in the literature are so similar to our own in clinical expression and pathological findings as to seem indeed carbon copies.

The significance of this identity is fairly obvious: It cannot be the result of a random process, but rather of a lesion in an identifiable vascular territory related to a recognizable clinical syndrome. In other words, the clinical features of these cases are related to a vascular lesion in much the same manner as Wallenberg's syndrome is related to posterior-inferior cerebellar artery occlusion or sylvian infarcts from the middle cerebral artery. This arterial territory related to akinetic mutism, which in the past has been vaguely referred to as "perforating branches from the posterior cerebral artery," "posterior thalamic vascular pedicle," or "retromammillary peduncle," has been recently identified by Percheron as the territory of the *posterior thalamosubthalamic paramedian artery.*

The following paragraphs give the profile of this new vascular syndrome. To date only 7 cases have been published with enough information to suit the purpose of this study.

One of the earlier reports is that of Bacaloglu, Raileanu, and Hornet

(1934), but their case was poorly studied from the clinical point of view, and the lesions were too widespread to allow precise localization, although parts of the reported infarct do indeed resemble the butterfly-shaped lesion of our study.

Another observation, by Brage, Morea, and Capello (1961), suffers from inadequate description of the pathological findings. One gains the impression, from sections reproduced of the hemispheres, that these patients did have the same kind of infarct as ours, but the study is too fragmentary to be useful.

Thompson's (1951) study is an important one. However, most of his patients had exceedingly extensive lesions which allow only approximate localizations. Only his Case 5 had two good coronal sections through the thalamus and mesencephalon showing the characteristic butterfly infarct. The clinical picture was that of "lethargic stupor" from which the patient could not be aroused even to speak.

French (1952) included 4 patients brought together because of the common trait of "prolonged unconsciousness." The extent of the lesions diminished the value of their topographic analysis. The author selected the mesencephalic tegmentum by the process of superimposing lesions from all cases, a procedure not without danger. His Cases 3 and 4 deserve mention, however. Case 3 was posttraumatic akinetic mutism, and the lesion responsible for it shared some of the territory supplied by the mesencephalic artery, suggesting a vascular factor in the production of the lesion. Case 4 is of great interest. This patient survived an episode of cardiac arrest, but remained akinetic and mute until he died. The interesting point is that the responsible lesions were situated in the *dorsal* thalamus, involving the dorsomedial nucleus (MD), anteriorventral nucleus (AV), ventralanterior nucleus (VA), ventrolateral nucleus (VL), and pulvinar, while the centrum medianum, the intralaminar and midline nuclei, and the cephalic portion of the mesencephalic tegmentum showed "surprisingly little alteration." In other words, the lesion was the reverse or negative copy of the responsible lesion in all the cases reported, even of French's other 3 cases. That the net clinical effect was the same is not too surprising: The deafferentation process postulated in the discussion below was carried out a step further up from the subthalamic area.

Angelergues, Ajuriaguerra, and Hécaen (1957) presented a patient whose infarct involved essentially the periventricular gray matter around the third ventricle and the periaqueductal gray matter in the area of the nuclei of Darkschewitsch and Cajal. This patient had a complex and interesting disturbance of eye movements, but no evidence of akinesia or mutism; in fact he was rather euphoric, excitable, and jocular. The lesion, however, was strictly periventricular and failed to extend laterally into the lower thalamus, leaving intact the reticulothalamic ascending systems. The thalamus in the patient was not disconnected from its reticular inputs.

Façon, Steriade, and Wertheim (1958) reported on a patient in whom the very tip of the basilar artery was occluded by a thrombus. The result was infarction of the calcarine cortex due to posterior cerebral insufficiency. In addition, however, a lesion germane to our study was present in the thalamosubthalamic area of both hemispheres on either side of the third ventricle. Clinically this 78-year-old woman was in a state of "sleep" for 3 years before death. Eye signs referred to the third cranial nerve were present, and this corresponded with the existence of infarction in the territory of the most inferior group of perforating arterioles branching from the mesencephalic artery. Rostral extension of the infarct near the anterior group of thalamic nuclei reflected the interference with the anterior perforating branch that Percheron has characterized so well (see below).

Castaigne *et al.* (1962) published another observation of atheromatous occlusion of the tip of the basilar artery. The result was a butterfly infarct destroying the midline and intralaminar nuclei, and the medial aspect of centrum medianum, and spreading laterally to the near vicinity of the ventroposterolateral (VPL) nucleus. A medial mesencephalic portion of the same infarct destroyed the third nerve nuclei, the medial longitudinal fasciculus (MLF), and part of the superior cerebellar peduncle. Clinically the most important symptom was hypersomnia, which persisted for 8 months until death.

Lhermitte *et al.* (1963) shortly afterward described another patient with nearly identical lesions. This 42-year-old woman became immobile and indifferent, unreactive to the surrounding world. After a while she became able to move her limbs, but only in response to vigorous entreaty and then only after long delays. She seemed "petrified" and was quite mute. Somnolence was an outstanding characteristic.

In a more recent report on this subject, Castaigne *et al.* (1966) referred to 2 cases which, because of the variations they present, deserve some comment. Lesions of the posterior thalamosubthalamic area were minimal, while the middle and anterior thalamic nuclear groups (MD, AV, etc.) had undergone extensive damage. The component of akinesia and mutism was relatively modest in these patients, while memory deficits and dementia were in the foreground. On the basis of Percheron's schema of vascular supply to this area, it seems reasonable to postulate an infarct in the territory of the *anterior* thalamosubthalamic paramedian artery. Both these cases illustrate another type of problem, i.e., dementias of thalamic origin, and will not be considered further.

Finally, Lechi and Macchi (1967) described a case of akinetic mutism occurring after encephalitis, with necrotizing lesions so similar to those in all the preceding studies as to suggest a vascular cause.

THE TERRITORY OF THE MESENCEPHALIC ARTERY

Students of the vascular system of the brain have generally considered the stretch of the posterior cerebral artery from the bifurcation of the basilar artery to the junction with the posterior communicating artery as a special vessel in itself. On embryological, morphological, and hemodynamic grounds this arterial segment should be set apart from the rest of the posterior cerebral artery. This segment is called the mesencephalic artery.

In the 52-day-old embryo (40 mm.) two branches arising from the rostral end of the basilar artery constitute the mesencephalic arteries (Kaplan and Ford, 1966). The posterior cerebral artery arises directly from the carotid artery. The initial stretch is referred to by most developmental anatomists as the "proximal portion" of the posterior cerebral artery and retains this name even after it becomes the posterior communicating artery. The "distal portion" refers to the stretch beginning at the junction with the mesencephalic artery and ending at the occipital pole. The mesencephalic artery arising from the tip of the basilar artery gives off a group of perforating branches before joining the posterior cerebral artery. After the junction, it goes around the brain stem like any other long circumferential vessel and supplies the colliculi.

The paramedian perforating branches of the mesencephalic artery are most interesting and relevant to our topic. They were studied by Foix and Hillemand (1925) as the "retromammillary pedicle" of the thalamic blood supply. They represent the most rostral group of all the perforating branches entering the brain in the posterior perforating space. Lazorthes (1961) found essentially a similar arrangement, but the most significant contribution in recent times is that of Percheron (1966), who systematized these vessels as follows:

1. Paramedian mesencephalic pedicle. This group penetrates the interpeduncular space giving off very few branches until terminal arborization around the oculomotor nuclei.

2. Thalamosubthalamic paramedian arteries. This group of branches is further divided in two subgroups with distinct arterial territories, namely, the anterior and the posterior. The posterior group (posterior thalamosubthalamic paramedian artery of Percheron) arises near the onset of the mesencephalic artery close to the midline. It penetrates the floor of the third ventricle and veers gently between the red nucleus below and the ventricular wall above. The vessel and its branches enter the thalamus at the level of the anterior pole of the centrum medianum. In all, it irrigates the medial-rostral part of the red nucleus and the subthalamic area above it, the posterior-inferior portion of the dorso-

medial nucleus (MD), the nucleus parafascicularis, the anterior and medial portions of the centrum medianum (CM), and perhaps some of the midline nuclei.

The perforating vascular systems so described have one important anatomical characteristic: The paramedian branches bifurcate near the midline in such a manner as to supply both hemispheres. The bilaterality of this territory corresponds nicely with the extent and disposition of the infarcts which are the object of this study.

MESENCEPHALIC AKINETIC MUTISM AND NEIGHBORHOOD SYMPTOMS

Given the anatomical complexity of the area, it is not surprising to find symptoms more or less closely associated with akinesia and mutism. Drowsiness is a common component of akinetic mutism. In contradistinction to the apathy of the patient with a cingulate or frontal lobe lesion (which, as Yakovlev has pointed out, is essentially a "wakeful" apathy), the patient with akinetic mutism of mesencephalic origin is often very sleepy. Hypersomnia and even disturbances in the sleep-wakefulness rhythm are often part of the syndrome.

Animal experimentation has shown how often both phenomena go together. The literature on the effect of upper brain-stem lesions on electroencephalographic, behavior, and sleep patterns in animals has grown to large proportions. The interested reader is referred to the work of French and Magoun (1952), Skultety (1962, 1965), and others. The net effect of this work is to show that lesions of the reticular formation of the mesencephalic tegmentum and the posterior-inferior portion of the medial thalamus can produce striking behavioral changes in the animal. Such changes consist of indifference, unreactivity, unresponsiveness, lethargy, helplessness, and mutism—all of which seems to agree with the clinical observation of the human subject.

Oculomotor disturbances of different kinds (pupillary asymmetries, third nerve paralysis, upward gaze paralysis, etc.) can be observed, and this is not surprising if one considers that the mesencephalic arterial pedicle arises from the mesencephalic artery at a point fairly close to the rostrally deviating thalamosubthalamic branches. Therefore, thrombosis at this level can shut off arterioles to the oculomotor nuclei as well as to the thalamus.

Dementia may be the result of rostral extension of the zone of infarct into the territory of the anterior-most branch of the mesencephalic artery, namely, the anterior thalamosubthalamic paramedian artery of Percheron, as was seen in the two cases reported by Castaigne *et al.* (1966).

It seems reasonable to attribute this syndrome of akinetic mutism to a differentiation or disconnection of midline and reticular thalamic structures from midline mesencephalic reticular formations. The lesion found in our cases and those of the literature interrupt reticulothalamic pathways as well as other fiber systems linking the midbrain to the limbic system, a fact which is not without theoretical interest.

Lesions of this kind interrupt most, if not all, of the ascending midbrain-limbic pathways (i.e., the ascending component of Schutz's dorsal longitudinal fasciculus, the mammillary peduncle, and the ascending component of the medial forebrain bundle) and they destroy descending limbic-midbrain fiber systems which, following Nauta and Whitlock (1954), may be listed as follows: (1) direct hippocampal projections from the fornix, (2) medial forebrain bundle, (3) mammillotegmental tract, (4) fasciculus retroflexus, and (5) the descending component of the dorsal longitudinal bundle of Schutz.

Lesions of slightly different distribution but in this general area have been shown by Denny-Brown (1962b) to produce, among other things, a profound apathy with indifference to the environment and an expressionless staring behavior, all elements, in part at least, of the akinetic state in humans.

As for the laterally situated lemniscal systems, it is doubtful what role, if any, they play in the production of akinetic mutism. The experimental work of Lindsley *et al.* (1950) showed that wakefulness and arousal responses are impaired after lesions of the medial core of the mesencephalic brain stem and, by contrast, remain undisturbed after lateral lesions destroying the lemnisci. It is not uncommon, moreover, to see human akinetic mutes reacting to painful and even tactile stimuli, something which can be accepted as qualified evidence of at least partially intact lemniscal systems.

There is little evidence for a "center of consciousness," but different aspects of what we call consciousness can be differentially affected through interruption of strategic pathways, not nuclei. It is precisely because of the nature of the lesion that one can expect changes in the clinical picture, since substitute pathways are usually available, although they may be less efficient.

CONCLUSIONS

1. Cerebrovascular disease, particularly ischemic infarction, is particularly suitable for the study of behavioral changes in man.

2. Careful pathological study, often involving serial sections of whole brain, of selected cases well studied clinically is the method of choice at the present time.

3. The minimal lesion responsible for akinetic mutism, as studied in 2 cases, is discussed, together with a review of the literature relevant to it.

4. The clinical picture of akinetic mutism of mesencephalic origin is due to occlusion of a perforating branch of the mesencephalic artery.

5. This branch has been recently identified as the posterior thalamo-subthalamic paramedian artery of Percheron. The territory of this vessel is bilateral and corresponds to the infarcts shown in our study.

6. It is proposed that this vascular infarct and its clinical expression be named the syndrome of the mesencephalic artery.

7. This territory includes the periventricular gray matter around the posterior portion of the third ventricle at the junction with the midbrain and extends laterally, butterfly-shaped, to affect the midline thalamic nuclei, the reticular nuclei of the thalamus, parafascicularis, and middle third of centrum medianum.

8. This review seems to indicate that akinetic mutism in these cases is due to a disconnection or deafferentation of thalamic nuclei from ascending midline mesencephalic reticular impulses.

PRESENTATION 2

John Moossy

The vague terms "cerebrovascular disease" and "behavior" will bedevil us throughout this workshop, and perhaps we deserve the torment. Segarra and Angelo have selected a particular clinical state, akinetic mutism, caused by a particular type of cerebrovascular disease, cerebral infarction. In attempting precision, they were unable to consider other alterations in human mental function which may be equally interesting to correlate with cerebrovascular disease. I will discuss certain aspects of their paper and call attention to some other areas of investigation.

Segarra and Angelo have spelled out the role of the neuropathologist. Adams (1959), in a thoughtful review of the contributions of the clinicopathological method to the study of human psychology, mentioned the role that cerebrovascular disease, among other disorders, has played in certain important cases. The neuropathologist indeed depends on detailed and accurate clinical information, since in most medical centers he is merely part of a team and the player who gets his chance last. Perhaps there is still a place for that vanishing type, the clinician-neuropathologist, who follows his patient clinically and does the pathoanatomical evaluation himself. Although we may feel a nostalgic urge (or moral responsibility) to cultivate and protect such individuals, current trends in medicine have repeatedly discouraged us.

Suitable cases for analysis must be accumulated; as Segarra and Angelo have stated, this may require much patience during the lean periods. Serendipity and a prepared mind are probably the most important factors in locating valuable case material. There is still a place for cautious speculation and hypothesis, even in cases which have not had ideal clinical evaluations. Some cases give us new clues too important to be ignored and they prepare us when better opportunities appear.

Serial sections of the whole brain are highly useful but not indispensable. Certain laboratories or special units within them should be supported in preparing serial sections. Only a few brains per year can be processed, and literally thousands of large slides must be cut, stained, and interpreted. It is to Dr. Segarra's credit that he has profited from the great contributions made by Yakovlev and his serial-section technique. I disagree that whole-brain serial sections are the *only* reliable means for study of the white matter; probably they are the best of several preparations and least likely to miss small tract and fascicular lesions. Secondary changes such as astrocytosis, retrograde and transneuronal degeneration, and wallerian degeneration add to the difficulties of interpretation no matter what technical methods are used. Electron microscopy, histochemistry, and quantitative neurochemistry may contribute additional information in selected cases without sacrificing the correlative value of standard techniques.

In spite of such obvious limitations as edema in the acute phase, cerebral infarcts and small hemorrhages may be especially appropriate for the study of anatomical-behavioral correlations. Cerebral infarcts lie in anatomically discrete vascular territories about which we have much scientific information, and therefore helpful comparisons are possible. Infarcts can be considered almost purely ablative or destructive lesions, although one cannot exclude some irritative component due to gliosis about the lesions in their later stages. These ablations due to infarction are more suitable for correlative studies than inflammatory, neoplastic, or traumatic lesions, which are usually more diffuse and are associated with edema and, in some instances, with mechanical distortions due to brain herniations. Similar objections apply to ruptured arterial aneurysms and bleeding vascular malformations. When the edema of the acute phase has subsided, usually in a few weeks, cerebral infarcts may be regarded as static ablative lesions which will produce deficit effects or "negative" signs. Infarcts can be roughly dated by their histopathological features so that in some instances strong inferences may be drawn about the clinical manifestations and the location of the responsible lesion even when there are multiple foci. Cases with embolic infarction, particularly with a solitary lesion, have yielded much valuable correlative information.

Akinetic mutism has been selected as a type of behavioral or psychomotor alteration to illustrate how small, discrete infarcts may result in profound impairment. Segarra and Angelo have advanced the definition of akinetic mutism by attempting a more precise classification. Their classification serves the pathologist better than the clinician, and distinctions are not always easy, especially among the conditions which they term apallic, cingulate, and mesencephalic states. An instructive illustration of these difficulties can be obtained by comparing the definitions of Segarra and Angelo with those in the recent review of akinetic mutism by Skultety (1968).

The arterial blood supply to the rostral mesencephalon and subthalamic-thalamic area is destined for a highly complex tissue. This neuroanatomical bottleneck is packed with the ascending reticular, lemniscal, and other pathways in close proximity to all tracts descending from the cerebral hemispheres. Little wonder then that small lesions in this area are capable of producing dramatic disorder. Segarra and Angelo have demonstrated more precisely localized, smaller lesions than in many cases reported in the literature. In spite of the sharper anatomical delineation in their cases, it is difficult to conclude with them that other patients with lesions in this area had strictly comparable changes in consciousness, vocalization, or kinesis. Now that Segarra and Angelo have documented this clinicopathological syndrome and produced some working definitions, additional cases can be more profitably compared with their own.

There are states other than akinetic mutism in which cerebrovascular disease has been or may be responsible for circumscribed lesions associated with distinctive psychological manifestations. Patients with well-defined atherosclerotic or embolic infarcts have been a source of valuable information in the study of aphasia, apraxia, and related higher cerebral functions. This is an old and well-known relationship of lesion and sign which will be explored in more detail in the papers by Geschwind, Joynt, and Spreen. Cerebrovascular disease, particularly infarction in the middle cerebral artery distribution, is often important in the pathogenesis of syndromes of the nondominant parietal lobe.

In a review of the role of the hippocampal-mammillary body complex in memory and memorizing, Barbizet (1963) did not mention cerebrovascular disease as an etiological factor in clinical illustrations of his hypothesis. Victor *et al.* (1961) presented a detailed clinicopathological study of a patient with a severe amnestic syndrome due to bilateral posterior cerebral artery occlusions and hippocampal infarcts. Recently De Jong, Itabashi and Olson (1968) reported another case of bilateral infarction of the parahippocampal gyri in which "pure" memory loss was the outstanding clinical feature. Vascular lesions, particularly infarcts, of the hippocampal complex and its connections will, and should, receive greater attention in the future.

The transient global amnesia syndrome is a peculiar clinical condition of current interest. First described by Bender (1956), then given its present name by Fisher and Adams (1964), this disorder almost exclusively affects older patients. Evans (1966) and Shuttleworth and Morris (1966) have reviewed the problem recently and reported additional cases. Although the pathogenesis has not been clarified, we are justified in suspecting a vascular factor, specifically cerebral vascular insufficiency, at least in some of the cases, because of the age of the patients and their associated vascular diseases. Small infarcts or merely transient, reversible, ischemic dysfunction in the hippocampal system might be suspected, but more study is necessary. No clinicopathological reports are yet available.

The importance of the tegmentum in vascular lesions of the pons was emphasized by Chase, Moretti and Prensky (1968) in their analysis of the clinical, electroencephalographic, and neuropathological features of 20 cases, 12 from the literature and 8 of their own. Their data supported the concept that bilateral tegmental lesions are necessary to abolish alertness and the electroencephalographic arousal response.

Finally I should refer briefly to dementia (or organic mental syndrome) due to cerebral arteriosclerosis alone, i.e., in the absence of multiple infarcts. Fisher (1968) appraised the problem at the Sixth Princeton Conference on Cerebrovascular Disease, and Millikan (1967), in a discussion of psychological reactions to aging, has called attention to the fact that such terms as "arteriosclerotic dementia" and "atherosclerotic degenerative brain disease" may be sources of confusion. While the issue has not been settled, the evidence to date suggests that chronic dementia of the elderly due to uncomplicated cerebral atherosclerosis alone is diagnosed more often than the data warrant. Some of the patients so diagnosed have multiple infarcts, some have degenerative neuronal disease of the Alzheimer senile dementia group and Jakob-Creutzfeldt disease, and some suffer from toxic metabolic disorders.

PRESENTATION 3

A. B. Baker
Manfred J. Meier

The detailed account provided by Segarra and Angelo of the vascular basis for a general behavioral state such as akinetic mutism requires no special comment. In a discussion of the pathological variables underlying behavioral change it seems appropriate to examine the pathophysiological basis of behavioral changes in cerebrovascular disease in the broader context of higher cortical functions and the adaptive implications of behavioral deficits associated with the more commonly encountered cerebrovascular episodes involving the internal carotid system. An exhaustive account of the many specific anatomical and related behavioral outcomes of cerebral infarcts would realistically be prohibitive. Therefore, the discussion which follows will emphasize some general pathophysiological considerations in cerebral atherosclerosis. In addition, a summary of recent behavioral findings associated with focal cerebral and subcortical lesions will be provided. Although most of the data on the relation between focal involvement and alterations in higher adaptive functioning were derived from focal involvement due to etiological variables unrelated to stenotic changes or thromboembolic events in the vessels, they may provide some anticipatory or predictive clues about the kinds of behavioral changes likely to occur in cerebrovascular disease.

GENERAL PATHOPHYSIOLOGICAL MODEL

Any attempt to correlate behavioral change with atherosclerotic changes in the extracranial and intracranial vessels would seem to proceed from the general assumption that behavioral change is determined by neuronal changes associated with cerebral ischemia or infarction. In support of this assumption, numerous arteriographic (Poser *et al.*, 1964) and autopsy (Martin, Whisnant, and Sayre, 1960; Millikan, 1967) studies have shown that extensive stenosis, including bilateral internal carotid occlusion and occlusion of both the carotid and vertebral basilar systems, is not unequivocally associated with cerebral infarction or conspicuous behavioral change. The necessary and sufficient pathophysiological condition underlying behavioral change, including focal neurological change, seems clearly to involve determinants which govern the maintenance of circulatory perfusion. Among these are included the relative site of the occlusion, the rate of development of the obstruction, the availability and amount of collateral circulation, and general systemic adequacy especially of the cardiovascular system (Toole and Patel, 1967). Resulting transient or permanent behavioral changes then depend upon the configuration of interacting pathophysiological events which produce reversible ischemia or irreversible infarction.

This general statement of the current pathophysiological model for behavioral change in cerebrovascular disease serves to underscore an obvious feature of the behavioral outcomes of transient ischemic attacks and cerebral infarctions. There does not appear to be a simple linear relation between changes in the vessels and behavioral or neurological changes. The inherent complexity of the pathophysiological events underlying neuropsychological changes makes such events difficult to anticipate or detect on a clinical or behavioral basis. The task of isolating and monitoring early pathophysiological changes in the symptom-free individual appears to be an incredibly complex undertaking. Before breakthroughs in the behavioral detection of early pathophysiological changes can be achieved, subtle behavioral deficits associated with small infarcts without focal neurological outcomes must be studied further.

The likely multivariate relation between behavior and cerebrovascular changes is succinctly highlighted by some paradoxical findings in a joint study of the natural history of stroke in Minnesota and in Kyushu, Japan (Meier and Okayama, 1966). As Meier has shown, performance on the Porteus Maze Test was much less impaired among patients with acute infarctions in Kyushu than in Minnesota. Differences on other measures in a neuropsychological test battery as well as in degree of rated clinical neurological involvement in this study implied less impairment of function among the Japanese after cerebrovascular occlusion. It seemed reasonable to consider differences in the pathophysiology of cerebral infarction between the two groups as a possible basis for a differential behavioral outcome. In this direction, four-vessel angiographic findings were analyzed for the two groups for all four vessels in the neck and their intracranial branches in two planes (Kieffer and Takeya, 1968). The Minnesota group exhibited greater frequency and severity of stenosis of the extracranial carotid circulation. On the other hand, the Japanese showed greater involvement of the intracranial portion of the internal carotid artery and of the anterior, middle, and posterior cerebral arteries. One implication of these data is that infarctions are likely to include more of the cerebral hemisphere in the Minnesota group, thus producing greater neurological and behavioral deficits. However, the differences on the Porteus Maze Test were present even when subgroups were matched for age, sex, lesion laterality, rated degree of neurological involvement, Wechsler Adult Intelligence Quotient, and time since symptom onset. Such an outcome appears to highlight the inherent complexity of pathophysiological determinants of behavior change, including individual and cultural factors which contribute to the organization of selected functions in the cerebral cortex. The mechanisms by which such differences in organization of cerebral function are generated may be multidimensional and nonlinear, involving culture-dependent learning conditions and/or genetic-racial factors.

REGIONAL LOCALIZATION OF HIGHER CORTICAL FUNCTIONS

It is beyond the scope of this paper to review extensively the evidence for the regional localization of behavioral functions in the brain. Excellent reviews of the major findings and methodological issues involved in the investigations of the behavioral correlates of focal brain lesions are available elsewhere (Meyer, 1960; Reitan, 1962; Piercy, 1964; Luria, 1966). Most of the behavioral research in this area has involved the assessment of sensorimotor, perceptual, and intellectual deficits and personality changes associated with focal cerebral lesions. Lesion location has been inferred on a clinical basis defined in terms of electrophysiological, angiographic, pneumoencephalographic, or scanning procedures and/or confirmed by means of neurosurgical intervention.

Many of these investigations have been concerned with establishing functional asymmetries between the cerebral hemispheres as assessed clinically and by means of neuropsychological testing methods. It has now been reasonably well established that the dominant cerebral hemisphere (the left hemisphere in individuals with right body-side preferences of usage) primarily subserves verbal intellectual functions, while the right (or nondominant) cerebral hemisphere mediates the integration of visuospatial and temporal-spatial relations. Thus the major behavioral correlate of structural lesions along the interhemispheric laterality dimension in man appears to involve differential changes in verbal and visuospatial functioning. In addition to interhemispheric asymmetries in function, the role of the corpus callosum in interhemispheric interaction has received considerable investigative attention in recent years (Mountcastle, 1962; Geschwind, 1965). The sections on language disturbances and objective behavioral assessment, later in this book, review much of this literature.

Similarly, higher-order behavioral changes have been observed to covary with the topographical location of focal lesions along the cephalocaudal dimension of the cerebral cortex. Rich but conflicting findings involving the behavioral effects of prefrontal lesions have not resolved earlier controversies over the functions of the prefrontal cortex. Although grossly quantitative reductions in general intelligence do not appear to occur after focal ablation or lobotomy(Mettler, 1949), there is growing evidence that declines in the integrity of purposive, goal-directed behavior consistently occur with lesions of the dorsolateral prefrontal cortex on either side (Milner, 1964; Luria, 1966). The related deficit appears to involve an impairment of autoregulation of purposeful motor behavior and is frequently characterized by perseveration, conceptual inflexibility, and faulty planning and foresight abilities. Such impairment seems most readily elicitable by means of tests which require sequenced motor behavior in a problem-solving situation like a paper-and-pencil maze (Porteus, 1955) and in sorting tasks involving a shift in the guiding principle in concept formation (Milner, 1964). Possible related deficits have been reported for rate of active scanning movements during prolonged examination of objects (Luria, 1966), setting a luminous line to the vertical under visuopostural conflict conditions (Teuber and Mishkin, 1954), executing instructions in a stylus-maze-learning situation (Milner, 1965), speed of visual search in the contralateral field in the absence of deficits in lateral gaze (Teuber, Battersby, and Bender, 1949), orientation to the body (Teuber, 1964), and temporal orientation (Benton, 1968a). In the context of cerebrovascular disease, such deficits might be expected to appear in the absence of general intellectual changes or persisting sensorimotor deficits. For example, selective occlusion of an anterior branch of the middle cerebral artery could produce an adaptively significant deficit of this kind without conspicuous focal neurological residuals. By contrast, cerebrovascular infarcts limited to the motor strip or situated deep in the white matter or internal capsule would be expected to produce profound sensorimotor deficits without changes in the goal-directed and planning components of problem-solving ability or in general intellectual functioning.

Although functional asymmetry of the prefrontal areas is not as great as that observed between the posterior regions of the cortex, selective impairment in word fluency has been observed after left prefrontal ablations involving the dorsolateral surface (Milner, 1964). Selectively, deficits in contralateral tactual pattern recognition, in the absence of somatosensory defects, have appeared after right frontal lobectomy (Milner, Taylor, and Corkin, 1967).

More recently, Benton (1968a) found that patients with left frontal lesions performed more poorly than patients with right frontal lesions on a measure of verbal associative fluency (Borkowski, Benton, and

Spreen, 1967), while patients with right frontal lesions showed greater deficits on a three-dimensional constructional task (Benton and Fogel, 1962; Benton, 1968b) and the copying version of the Visual Retention Test (Benton, 1962).

Most of the deficits arising from prefrontal lesions are as yet incompletely understood. As will be discussed below, a motivational component in the impulsive behavior predispositions underlying the most characteristic deficit could well result from disruptions in the anatomical-physiological interactions between portions of the frontal lobe and the limbic system.

Lesions of the posterior regions of the cerebral cortex appear to produce greater intellectual impairment than do lesions in the frontal lobes, particularly with dominant hemisphere involvement (Weinstein, 1962). Interhemisphere differentiation in function also seems more prevalent in posterior temporal-parietal cortex where well-known and sometimes profound changes in perceptual and intellectual function have been well documented (Teuber, 1959; Meyer, 1960; Piercy, 1964; Luria, 1966). Examination of the research literature reveals considerable convergence of the classical clinical neurological and the more formal objective neuropsychological approaches.

Substantial reviews of the clinical literature, along with prevalence data for aphasic, apraxic, somatagnosic, and visuospatial agnostic disturbances as a function of lesion location are now available (Hécaen, 1962; Luria, 1966). Recent attempts to combine the methodology of the clinical neurological and neuropsychological testing approaches provide promise of an interdisciplinary consolidation of knowledge in this area of inquiry. These attempts are noteworthy in the present context insofar as the samples studied have included sizable numbers of patients with cerebrovascular occlusive disease (Arrigoni and De Renzi, 1964; De Renzi and Faglioni, 1965, 1967; De Renzi, Pieczuro, and Vignolo, 1966, 1968). Since much of this work is discussed in other papers in this volume, the remainder of this presentation will be limited to some recent findings which bear upon the functions of the anterior temporal lobe and the role of the deeper limbic and subcortical structures in the mediation of behavior.

Data relative to the behavioral effects of anterior temporal lobectomy have consistently suggested certain functional asymmetries between the temporal lobes. In contrast to lateralized posterior temporal-parietal lesions, however, anterior temporal lobe involvement has produced behavioral changes which are clinically less conspicuous and somewhat difficult to elicit. Specialized testing procedures have revealed that the anterior temporal lobe contributes to verbal learning, memory, and perceptual processes, with the kind of deficit depending upon lesion laterality and the particular structures involved.

Patients characteristically exhibit impairment of verbal learning and verbal memory after removal of the left anterior temporal lobe even in the absence of gross dysphasic changes (Meyer and Yates, 1955; Milner and Kimura, 1964). Deficits on verbal tasks in such patients are observed irrespective of how memory functioning is measured or of the sensory channel utilized. Although the deficits are present preoperatively, significantly more impairment results from removal of the temporal lobe. Perceptual processing of information fed into the two ears by the technique of Broadbent (1954), in which different digits are presented simultaneously, is only mildly impaired, so that the characteristic verbal loss after left temporal lobectomy apparently transcends immediate memory span and the perception of stimuli. This is especially demonstrable when the testing involves a 1-hour delay between initial reading and recall of short prose passages; in this situation, patients with left temporal lobectomy show more severe retention losses than groups with other focal lesions (Milner, 1958, 1964). The deficit appears also to be related to the extent and kind of tissue removal. Preliminary indications that functional interaction between the hippocampus and the temporal neocortex are involved in verbal memory functioning are currently being explored (Milner, 1967). Functional relations between the hippocampus and temporal neocortex may also prove to subserve the transfer of symbolic learning from one hand to the other. For example, Meier and French (1965a) have reported a selective deficit with the right hand after learning with the left hand on an inverted alphabet printing task in patients with left, as compared with right, temporal lobe ablations. In addition to transfer of learning, it may be that cortical inhibition, accumulated through habituation in repetitive learning tasks, dissipates less rapidly in verbal learning situations after left, and in nonverbal learning after right, temporal lobe lesions, especially if interrelations between the temporal lobe and the information-storage mechanism of the hippocampus have been disrupted by the lesion. Such effects could significantly impair the residual adaptive capacity of patients with highly circumscribed infarcts critically located in this region even if general intellectual function and sensorimotor status remain intact.

Right temporal lobectomy has been associated with impairment of the ability to (1) recognize irregular patterned stimuli (Kimura, 1963); (2) sequentially organized complex pictorial stimuli (Milner, 1958; Meier and French, 1966a); (3) discriminate fragmented concentric circular patterns (Meier and French, 1965a); and (4) recall faces (Milner, 1958) and unfamiliar nonsense figures (Kimura, 1963). These losses are similar to the visual discrimination deficits produced in monkeys after bilateral excision of the inferior temporal cortex (Chow, 1950; Mishkin and Pribram, 1954) and support the view that the temporal lobes provide an extrastriate focus for visually guided behavior which, in man, appears to be differentiated on a lateral basis. Similar deficits in audition have been observed after right anterior lobectomy on various subtests of the Seashore Measures of Musical Talents (Saetveit, Lewis, and Seashore, 1940) involving the discrimination of tonal patterns, tone quality or timbre, and tonal memory (Milner, 1962). These deficits are relatively permanent and are not contingent upon removal of the primary auditory projection cortex (Milner, 1967).

Visual and tactual stylus-maze-learning deficits have appeared after right anterior temporal lobectomy (Milner, 1965; Corkin, 1965), although the Porteus Maze Test failed to differentiate right from left temporal lobectomized patients (Meier and French, 1966a). The importance of deeper structures in generating such deficits is indicated by the fact that the emergence of the stylus-maze-learning deficit after right temporal removals appears to require destruction of the hippocampus (Milner, 1967). In addition, stereotaxic lesions placed in the subthalamic region of the field of Forel have consistently produced a decline after right but not after left, subthalamotomy (Meier and Story, 1967). As in the findings reported by Segarra and Angelo, highly circumscribed subthalamic lesions can produce extensive behavioral alterations. The findings of Meier and Story seem to imply that lesions in areas such as the field of Forel with rich connections to specific thalamic nuclei and to limbic and/or midbrain structures can interrupt functions subserved by a corresponding region of the cerebral cortex. Such a formulation would be compatible with the growing body of anatomical and physiological evidence for ascending organization of structure and function in the central nervous system (Magoun, 1958). The more generalized behavioral changes associated with bilaterally symmetrical vascular lesions of the thalamomesencephalic junction described by Segarra and Angelo are analogous to these changes as well as to the profound disruption of the cerebral organization of memory observed after bilateral destruction of the hippocampus (Milner, 1967).

Further evidence for the development of more generalized behavioral disturbances with bilateral central nervous system involvement can be derived from studies of personality change and focal lesions and ablations. The interaction between anatomical and physiological systems organized along the vertical axis of the central nervous system structure has been recognized to be of fundamental importance in the functional organization of emotional and motivational patterns of behavior in animals (Klüver and Bucy, 1938; Bard and Mountcastle, 1948; MacLean and Delgado, 1953; Brady, 1958; Olds, 1958; Ruch, 1961). Anatomically, it has become apparent that efferent projections from the hippocampus and cingulate cortex lead to the midbrain reticular formation which interconnects reciprocally with the nonspecific intralaminar nuclei of the thalamus (Johnson, 1953). These nuclei have been shown to interact anatomically with limbic system structures in an ascending and descending manner (Nauta, 1953, 1956) and, along with the midbrain reticular formation, project to the neocortex (Morison and Dempsey, 1942; Moruzzi and Magoun, 1949). Moreover, the limbic system, in addition to the temporal pole and deeper subcortical structures, includes portions of the frontal lobe, specifically the orbital frontal surface and the cingulate cortex (Ramón y Cajal, 1909; Lorente de Nó, 1934). This system, therefore includes both frontal and temporal components, as well as the hippocampus, amygdala, and insula, to form a vertically organized system whose complex interrelations are maintained through the uncinate fasciculus (Kendrick and Gibbs, 1958).

In this context, there is some preliminary evidence that selected personality changes in man, as measured by the Minnesota Multiphasic Personality Inventory (MMPI), occur with limbic system involvement (Meier and French, 1964a,b; 1965b). Bilateral electroencephalographic abnormalities, especially bitemporal independent spike foci, are associated with greater MMPI indications of schizoadaptive behavioral alterations than are unilateral electroencephalographic abnormalities. These personality characteristics, as judged from the scale items, include anxiety, depression, guilt feelings, social withdrawal, feelings of inadequacy and isolation, somatic concern, schizoid interpersonal adjustment, and schizophrenic-like ideational disturbances. These findings suggest that intrinsic pathophysiological variables affecting limbic system function contribute to personality change. MMPI scale reductions observed after neurosurgical removal of the primary pathophysiologically discharging focus, particularly in patients with bitemporal electroencephalographic spike foci, are consistent with a direct causal relation between a discharging focus in the limbic system and personality disturbances.

This treatment of some recent behavioral findings implicating various central nervous system structures is not intended to be exhaustive. Emphasis has been placed on data regarding the effects of lesions in areas whose functions have been difficult to assess. This was done on the assumption that such behavioral changes might provide a basis in the future for detecting cerebrovascular ischemia or infarction in the absence of focal neurological changes. As a supplement to the presentation of Segarra and Angelo, our purpose has been to add emphasis to the role of subcortical as well as cortical pathophysiological factors in the generation of behavioral changes.

SECTION II

Language Disturbances in Cerebrovascular Disease

PRESENTATION 4

Norman Geschwind

A skeptical reader might well ask whether there is any reason to devote attention to the language disturbances of cerebrovascular disease rather than to treat the more general topic of language disturbances resulting from cerebral disease without regard to etiology. It has indeed long been a cliché of clinical neurology that it is localization rather than pathology which determines the pattern of functional derangement. Although this venerable teaching is generally correct, it neglects certain important considerations such as the time over which a lesion develops which may in fact profoundly affect its outward manifestations. As will be shown, there are both theoretical and practical considerations which must lead us to a discussion of aphasic syndromes consequent upon disease of the blood vessels of the brain.

Before proceeding further, let us first specify the kinds of cerebrovascular diseases with which we will be dealing. When we speak of behavioral change with cerebrovascular disease, we are concerned overwhelmingly with the effects of ischemic infarction, primarily as a result of thrombosis and to a lesser degree from embolism. Because of the generally poor prognosis of primary cerebral hemorrhage, it is a relatively minor cause of permanent aphasias. Cerebral aneurysm plays a small role in comparison with thrombosis as a cause of language disturbances. In its occasional function as a space-occupying mass the aneurysm is a rare cause of aphasia. Insofar as it leads to focal signs resulting either from intracerebral rupture or from secondary ischemia, its effects are similar to those of primary hemorrhage or infarction. The therapy of aneurysms has, in the experience of our aphasia center, been a not infrequent cause of aphasia in patients referred from a broad area. Carotid ligation, when followed by right hemiplegia, is often accompanied by aphasia, while direct surgical treatment of an aneurysm may lead to aphasia particularly when extensive dissection is required in the left temporal lobe. Progressive dementia or akinetic mutism following aneurysm rupture, often the result of communicating hydrocephalus (frequently with normal cerebrospinal fluid pressure), are important behavioral syndromes, but not of direct concern to the problem with which we are dealing. These conditions are of some interest in differential diagnosis in that occasionally a patient with akinetic mutism is misdiagnosed as aphasic. Similarly, the error is occasionally made of diagnosing as aphasic the patient who is in a state of acute confusion following aneurysm rupture.

A related problem should be mentioned briefly, i.e., the aphasic syndromes resulting as a complication of arteriography for the investigation of cerebrovascular disease. These do not differ in principle from aphasias caused by other acute occlusive diseases.

IMPORTANCE OF THE APHASIAS FOLLOWING STROKE

We may discuss the importance of these aphasias under several headings: social, diagnostic, and theoretical. The social problem of aphasia is a major one, and indeed it is probably the most important type of behavioral disturbance resulting directly from cerebrovascular disease. For a large number of patients it is the sole disability resulting from stroke and for many others the most crippling, often being the only factor preventing useful adjustment. Despite these facts, it is curious that we have very little precise knowledge of the magnitude of the problem. We know the number of patients dying of stroke in any given year, but we have by contrast little idea of how many aphasic patients there are in the United States. Similarly, we have only spotty information about the social arrangements under which these patients live or what becomes of them. The possession of such knowledge would be useful for any future plans for dealing with the consequences of stroke.

From the theoretical view, it is important to stress that it is the patient with the chronic ischemic infarct who is the most important source of knowledge concerning the clinical syndromes of the aphasias and their localizations. Thrombotic cerebrovascular disease is by far the most important cause of aphasia in the adult. These patients can be studied over long periods of stability. At postmortem examination the lesions found are often well defined and can be mapped precisely, together with the resultant secondary degenerations.

There are, of course, many patients, the study of whose brains may provide us with little information. All too frequently clinical study in life has been inadequate. The brain at autopsy may contain multiple lesions which prevent useful correlation. Despite these difficulties, a significant number of cases are seen which meet all the requirements for proper study. Tumor material is less well suited to this kind of investigation. Distortion of the brain or the infiltrating character of the neoplasm may make impossible specification of the extent of the lesion. Effects at a distance through pressure, vascular changes, or edema provide further impediments to precise correlative studies. Cortical excisions for epilepsy are highly useful, but in general they give information about patients with lesions of early onset who have suffered many seizures and who thus represent a special population from whom it may be difficult to draw conclusions concerning adult aphasics.

We can appreciate even more the importance of the stroke-induced aphasias when we realize that the paucity of examples of certain vascular lesions has seriously hampered the study of many nonaphasic disturbances of the higher functions. Patients with vascular lesions of the frontal regions on either side are scarce, as are patients with vascular lesions of the right hemisphere not producing hemiplegias, e.g., right frontal (nonmotor), right temporal, and right parietal lesions. As a result, many published series compare patients with aphasia, often the result of vascular disease, and patients with right hemisphere lesions which are most commonly tumors. This divergence of pathological substrates compromises the validity of conclusions concerning the differential effects of right and left hemisphere lesions. One might parenthetically inquire why there is a paucity in clinical practice of patients with right hemisphere vascular lesions in the absence of hemiplegia. Descriptions in the literature of the syndromes of infarction of these regions in the absence of hemiplegia are rare. We could perhaps surmise that in the early stage many of these patients present acute confusional states, while in the later stage they present syndromes capable of being elicited only by subtle testing techniques. Perhaps the increased use of radioactive scanning will permit greater recognition of such patients and will aid in filling important lacunae in our knowledge.

Investigation of vascular lesions also represents almost the only way, although certainly not an ideal one, to study in man the effects of certain lesions which produce transient syndromes. In animals certain lesions produce syndromes which disappear in 1 or 2 weeks, e.g., the remarkable syndrome of contralateral inattention resulting from unilateral frontal lesions, described by Kennard (1939) and more recently by Welch and Stuteville (1958). In man excisions are never carried out in normal areas of normal brains, and the only equivalent situation is the acute vascular insult. A well-known example in man is the conjugate gaze difficulty following damage to the frontal eye fields, which occurs transiently in association with vascular disease. Tumors rarely produce this syndrome, since the compensation which develops slowly after a stroke takes place during the growth of a space-occupying tumor. Transient aphasias after lesions of the supplementary motor area probably represent a similar situation. We suspect strongly that premotor lesions may cause transient unilateral inattention syndromes in man (and may indeed be the most common cause of such syndromes), just as they do in animals. Seizures, of course, may also produce transient syndromes, but these are usually of even shorter duration than those after destructive lesions and are thus even more difficult to study.

It is important to recognize that certain types of chronic aphasic syndrome may be seen in cerebrovascular disease but are rarely observed as the sequel of other kinds of pathology. Thus nearly all cases of permanent pure alexia without agraphia are the result of cerebrovascular disease (Geschwind, 1962). The reason for this is that the usual pathology, i.e., the combination of destructive lesions involving both the left calcarine cortex and the splenium of the corpus callosum, is highly unlikely as a result of tumor, surgery, or penetrating wounds of the brain. The recognition that certain aphasic symptoms occur rarely except as the result of vascular disease is often useful diagnostically. Thus Alzheimer's disease, while commonly causing some type of aphasia, almost never leads to certain specific syndromes, e.g., to the classical Broca's aphasia, conduction aphasia, or pure alexia without agraphia. The presence of any of these in a patient, at least in the early stages, would almost certainly exclude the diagnosis of Alzheimer's disease.

APHASIAS IN CEREBROVASCULAR DISEASE

We will discuss briefly some of the aphasic syndromes with stress on their vascular origins.

TRANSIENT APHASIAS

Aphasias in cerebrovascular disease may be transient for two reasons: (1) the lesion may not be destructive, as in transient ischemic attacks, and (2) the lesion may be destructive but the effects transient. For example, the evidence suggests that destruction of the supplementary motor area may lead to transient aphasia (Penfield and Roberts, 1959), a situation which should be suspected when aphasia is accompanied by signs of a right hemiplegia worse in the leg, i.e., the hemiplegic syndrome characteristic of anterior cerebral artery occlusion. A similar transient syndrome is the defect in acquisition of new knowledge, which may last even up to 3 months after infarction of the left hippocampal region by an occlusion of the posterior cerebral artery (Geschwind and Fusillo, 1966). We should distinguish those destructive lesions which nearly always produce transient syndromes (e.g., those involving frontal eye fields, supplementary motor area, or left hippocampal region) from those in which transiency is not the rule but occurs occasionally. Thus while some aphasics remain unchanged for years, others may improve over long periods of time, in some cases even to normal, probably as a result of increasing right hemisphere participation in speech functions.

APHASIC SYNDROMES RESULTING FROM DAMAGE TO SPECIFIC VESSELS

Anterior Cerebral Artery. Lesions of this vessel rarely cause aphasia, but they may in the following circumstances:

1. After destruction of the supplementary motor area, transient aphasia may occur (see above).
2. If the anterior four-fifths of the callosum is infarcted, aphasia may result if there is a previous or accompanying lesion of the left internal capsule, thus cutting off both the normal outflow pathway for speech from the left hemisphere and the alternative route over the corpus callosum (Bonhoeffer, 1914).

Middle Cerebral Artery. Probably the great majority of aphasias result from lesions in the distribution of this vessel.

1. *Global aphasia,* the syndrome produced by destruction of both Broca's and Wernicke's areas, results from infarctions of the entire opercular region. It is nearly always accompanied by severe hemiplegia. More limited lesions affecting regions within the middle cerebral distribution produce more delimited syndromes.
2. *Broca's aphasia* results from a lesion involving the posterior portion of the frontal operculum, which may be either cortical or subcortical, effectively undercutting this region. The vascular lesions producing this picture are almost invariably large enough to produce an accompanying hemiplegia worse in the arm.
3. *Wernicke's aphasia* is produced by a lesion involving the posterior-superior temporal region. Hemiplegias are usually not present.
4. *Conduction aphasia* results from a lesion involving the anterior-inferior parietal region. It may be accompanied by a parietal sensory loss on the right side. I have seen a case in which this was accompanied by a thalamic syndrome, probably also the result of a lesion of the parietal operculum, such as was described by Biemond (1956).
5. *Pure word deafness* results from a lesion deep in the temporal lobe. There is usually little other disability.
6. *Anomic aphasia* is produced by a lesion in the angular gyrus.
7. *Pure alexia with agraphia* results from an angular gyrus lesion. It is sometimes accompanied by hemianopia if the lesion goes deep to the ventricle, thus cutting the optic radiations.

Posterior Cerebral Artery. The one common aphasic syndrome from lesions within the distribution of this vessel is *pure alexia without agraphia,* in which the infarct involves the left calcarine cortex plus the splenium of the corpus callosum. Almost all permanent cases of this syndrome are the result of cerebrovascular disease.

Watershed Areas. Syndromes of great vessel insufficiency may produce distinctive effects because of their tendency to produce infarcts at the border zones between the middle cerebral arterial region and the regions of the posterior and anterior cerebral arteries. These lesions often cut through the angular gyrus and produce some of the syndromes already mentioned. The most dramatic aphasic syndrome of this type is, however, the one which results when the border zone infarct produces a large C-shaped lesion surrounding the language areas, which are left intact, but isolated. This is called the *syndrome of the isolated speech area* and may be produced by ischemia, hypoxia, or hypoglycemia but rarely results from other causes (Geschwind, Quadfasel, and Segarra, 1968).

EMOTIONAL CHANGES WITH APHASIA

Since this workshop deals with the broad topic of behavioral changes in cerebrovascular disease, it is appropriate to discuss here some of the characteristic behavioral alterations which occur in the stroke-induced aphasias. It is important to distinguish here, as in all cases of emotional change after brain lesions, those which are the effects of response to stress and those which are more intimately related to the site of the lesion in the central nervous system. Thus a patient with paraplegia following ischemia of the cord would be expected to respond in much the same way as a patient who has undergone a sudden amputation. Certain brain lesions, on the other hand, produce syndromes dependent on their own localization and physiology.

The patient with classical Broca's aphasia characteristically responds to the sudden onset of his disability in a way that appears appropriate. He is typically depressed and often tearful. He weeps when he is reassured by the doctor; he is distressed at his own errors in testing. The fluent aphasic is on the whole less disturbed by his own disabilities, but even this lack of fully normal response varies by diagnostic category. Thus patients with conduction and with anomic aphasia are usually aware of and distressed by their errors, but are usually not as depressed as those with Broca's aphasia. The usual lack of severe hemiplegia in these cases may perhaps contribute to this difference in response.

The patient with Wernicke's aphasia, by contrast, generally appears quite unaware of his disturbance and indeed is frequently euphoric. If he shows personality change, it is often in the direction of becoming angry with those around him. The essential reason for this difference is, of course, that he lacks the *internal* mechanisms to monitor his own speech output.

The patient with pure word deafness stands in sharp contrast to the one with Wernicke's aphasia despite the apparent similarity of their lack of comprehension of speech. Typically the word-deaf patient complains bitterly. A feature of the patient with pure word deafness found in early clinical descriptions, and one that our own experience has verified, is a tendency to become increasingly paranoid. The patient with pure alexia tends to be fully aware of his deficits, but unable to understand the discrepancy between his ability to see and to read.

The patient with Wernicke's aphasia can present the most dramatic psychiatric syndromes. As we have noted, euphoria is common, but marked agitation and anger may become increasingly difficult to manage. It has been our experience that nearly all patients who required transfer from our aphasia unit to the psychiatric service had Wernicke's aphasia. Sometimes agitation and anger appear at the onset, and the sudden appearance of these combined with bizarre speech and the usual absence of elementary neurological signs may lead to an incorrect diagnosis of an acute psychiatric state, a point first mentioned by Wernicke (1874) himself and later repeated by Adolf Meyer (1909–1910).

METHODS OF STUDY IN LIFE

We will not discuss pathological investigation, since this has been dealt with by other contributors to this volume. One of the great problems in the study of aphasia has been the paucity of adequate methods for obtaining further information concerning the sites of the lesions in the living patient. Several techniques are now available that can contribute to further knowledge of these syndromes.

1. *Intracarotid Amytal studies* (Wada test), at present included in only a minor fraction of the many arteriographic studies performed, should be carried out in cases of aphasia resulting from cerebrovascular disease. They would be particularly valuable in cases of recovery from, or alteration of, the clinical picture of aphasia after left-sided lesions to determine the extent to which right-hemisphere substitution plays a role in such changes.

2. The *Broadbent* (1954) *technique*, which was brilliantly applied to the study of brain lesions by Kimura (1967), has been primarily used following removal of the temporal pole or cortical excision in pa-

tients with epilepsy. The technique deserves further application to determine the effects of other types of lesions, especially those in regions not likely to be damaged by the surgeon. Correlation of these findings with lesions seen postmortem may help to define further the pathways involved in dichotic listening.

3. *Radioactive scanning* has been of great value in our hands in the study of the aphasias resulting from cerebrovascular disease. Benson and Patten (1967) have made several studies of the correlations between the clinical localizations and the scan abnormalities of patients in our aphasia unit. We have found that the second week is the ideal period for this study. The slow, but high-resolution, techniques are excellent for this purpose.

4. Another technique, described for some years, but only recently applied by us to the problem of localization of aphasia-producing lesions, deserves mention here. It was called to our attention by Dr. Cesare Lombroso. The patient is given pentothal intravenously while the electroencephalogram is being recorded. We use special electrode placements to bracket the sylvian region more carefully. This technique relies on the absence of the usual electroencephalographic signs of barbiturate effect in the damaged areas.

SUMMARY

The aphasias resulting from cerebral infarction are probably the most common behavioral consequence of cerebrovascular disease and thus have great social importance. They also have diagnostic and theoretical importance. Certain aphasic syndromes, both transient and permanent, are rarely seen except as a result of stroke. In addition, the permanent aphasic syndromes following cerebral infarction are the most useful source of information concerning localization of the causative lesion.

The transient and permanent aphasic syndromes associated with damage to the cerebral arteries and watershed areas are reviewed. Techniques which permit localizing information to be obtained in life are also discussed briefly.

PRESENTATION 5

Robert J. Joynt

Geschwind has asked whether the language disturbances seen with cerebrovascular disease should be considered apart from disturbances due to other causes. He has answered his own question largely by pointing out that certain aphasic disturbances are seen almost exclusively with vascular disease and that the stability of the lesions makes them particularly suitable for long-term study and anatomical-clinical correlation.

I will mention two aspects of this problem which were alluded to by Geschwind and which point out some other singular features about language disturbances arising from cerebrovascular lesions. It is, as pointed out, a neurological verity that the location rather than the process determines the functional deficit. But there are two other elements which, while not abrogating, do complicate this venerable rule: (1) the "momentum" or the length of time over which a lesion develops, and (2) the nature of the lesion.

EFFECT OF MOMENTUM OF LESION

The complicating features of these elements are best brought out in cerebrovascular disease, and particularly in considering the language disturbances associated with vascular lesions. The effect of momentum is evident in the common clinical observation that the aphasic disturbance, or disorder of any other cerebral function, is much more severe after a sudden lesion such as a stroke than after a slowly developing one such as a tumor, when both lesions are comparable in terms of location and extent of brain involvement as determined during life by various diagnostic procedures and after death by pathological examination.

The influence of rapidity of damage on brain function was mentioned briefly by Marc Dax in 1836. When speaking of language representation in the left hemisphere, Dax noted: "I would not even regard as an exception a disease of the left hemisphere without alteration of speech, particularly if the disease were slight or if it had developed slowly." (Cited by Joynt and Benton, 1964.) It was discussed several times by Hughlings Jackson, and the term "momentum of lesion" was first used by him in 1879. He occasionally, in his arcane literary style, used the physicists' designation, *mv* (mass × velocity), for this. He pointed out: "In all cases of nervous disease we must endeavor to estimate most carefully the element of rapidity of lesions, not only the quantity of nervous elements destroyed, but the rapidity of their destruction. We have to try to estimate the momentum of lesions. . . . A small sudden hemorrhage produces greater but a more temporary effect, provided it does not at once kill, than a large, slowly developed softening." Jackson (1894) later stated this as a doctrine, saying: "The more rapidly the dissolution is effected the greater is the activity on the range of evolution remaining."

The finding that functional disturbance may reflect something more than structural change was central to Von Monakow's (1914) doctrine of "diaschisis." It is in cerebrovascular lesions that we usually encounter this phenomenon. Von Monakow looked upon this as a suspension of activity of those parts having neural connections with the local lesion, i.e., functionally separated—hence, his term meaning to split apart. Von Monakow (1911) emphasized disparity between lesion and functional deficit as follows: "No matter how the further investigation may turn out, I am convinced by our latest studies of functional dissolution that diaschisis or some similar consideration cannot be neglected. Diaschisis represents, in association with other forms of shock, a dynamic basic principle, for it creates a bridge between a nervous phenomenon which is distinctly and precisely localized and one which is not."

The importance of the effect of evolution of a lesion was emphasized by Riese (1948) in a study of 5 patients with similarly located lesions evolving with varying rapidity. He found the degree of aphasic disturbance closely related to the rapidity of development, and concluded: "Sudden lesions, i.e., those of greatest momentum, are most likely to produce aphasia, though only transitory in uncomplicated cases. In lesions of slow momentum, speech may be preserved either throughout the whole history, or, at least, for a long time."

This widespread disruption of function from a localized lesion has not been totally explained. It is seen clinically when, for example, bilateral signs are present after a sudden infarct of one hemisphere. There is also a disruption in the electrical activity of the brain as seen in the common electroencephalographic finding of bilateral changes after a unilateral cerebral infarct. Various theories have been adduced: generalized vasospasm following a stroke, secondary transneuronal inactivation of brain tissue with consequent reduced cerebral blood because of decreased metabolic demands, and the phenomenon of spreading depression. Kempinsky (1966) points out that none of these are entirely satisfactory explanations.

Cerebrovascular lesions by their rapid evolution do present singular clinical features which may complicate our problem of anatomical-clinical correlation. An aphasic disturbance may represent functional derangement of a large area of brain disrupted by a small lesion, and indeed the inciting local lesion may be distant from those areas involved in language function. Obviously, the pathologist's dissection gives us no information about functional disruption in the face of intact structure.

EFFECT OF NATURE OF LESION

The relation of the nature of the lesion to the severity of language disturbance is emphasized by considering the deficit after strokes compared with that associated with brain tumors of glial origin (the most common type). Consideration of only the location, and not the nature of the lesion may lead to confusion, since studies of anatomical-functional correlation are often based on a series composed of patients with tumors and patients with vascular lesions. Strokes (thrombotic lesions) wreak their devastation by ischemia and thus affect neural tissue prior to supporting tissue. This is due, of course, to the marked sensitivity of neurons and the relative resistance of glia to oxygen and substrate deficit. Tumors, however, arise from the glial tissue and may, even when far advanced, leave functional neural tissue intact—the tumor insinuating itself between nerve cells and tracts. This accounts for the common clinical observation that patients are usually much worse after tumor removal, as still-functioning neural tissue must necessarily be excised. Thus, infarcts and tumors of comparable size and location as determined by the usual diagnostic tests may have a much different impact on brain function.

SUMMARY

Both the momentum and the nature of the lesion must be considered, in addition to its location, when clinical-anatomical correlations are made. That these factors are often neglected may account for some of the disparate analyses of brain-behavior dysfunction. It is particularly important that we take note of these factors in studying language dysfunction following cerebrovascular lesions.

PRESENTATION 6

Otfried Spreen

In his introduction to this section, Geschwind has outlined the aphasic syndromes found predominantly in patients with cerebrovascular disease. He has also made a case for treating the aphasias in cerebrovascular disease separately and independently of the aphasias of different etiology. If it can be shown that certain aphasic syndromes occur predominantly or exclusively with specific cerebrovascular lesions, then the diagnostic, prognostic, and therapeutic implications of these findings cannot be overestimated.

In this discussion I will not try to elaborate on Geschwind's survey. Instead, I will concentrate on two methodological problems: (1) the problem of classifying the aphasias, particularly aphasias following cerebrovascular lesions, and (2) the problem of assessing behavioral changes. I will also comment on Geschwind's remarks about pure alexia without agraphia.

Geschwind's survey has used the traditional nomenclature of the aphasias based on the experience of clinicians for the past 100 years. The terminology has naturally emerged from numerous study reports covering one or several well-selected cases. This case study method is still the predominant approach. Large-scale studies are quite rare. A brief review of the literature pertaining to cerebrovascular disease found several studies based on large numbers of patients (e.g., Gurdjian *et al.*, 1960), but the aphasic syndromes in such patients were either neglected or treated in gross summary fashion. If we are to accept a classification system such as the one presented by Geschwind for the aphasic syndromes in cerebrovascular disease and if we are to assess the clinical, sociological, and prognostic importance of these syndromes, then we should attempt the detailed evaluation of large series of patients.

Geschwind has commented upon the lack of long-term follow-up studies of patients with aphasia, and the findings in the few individual cases that have been followed for long periods emphasize the need for careful and detailed study. For example, some patients make only an apparently satisfactory adjustment, as did a man in his fifties who managed for years to run his small electrical contracting and appliance shop in spite of fairly severe motor aphasia and right hemiparesis. This seemed to indicate good adjustment in the presence of severe handicap. Closer investigation, however, revealed that he managed his shop only with the active help of his wife and a senior employee; that his relation with these loyal helpers was stressed by occasional paranoic trends in his behavior, and that his business was on a downhill course. Other patients show a striking true recovery, as did a young lady who 1 year after an ischemic episode with severe aphasia managed to regain and hold a job as an operator for the local telephone company. Many patients with global aphasia seem to change from an initial euphoric state to a depressive one before adjusting to a more normal emotional level. Improvement of the aphasia apparently does not begin until the patient reaches the depressive phase in which he is able to recognize his own errors and make serious attempts to cooperate during therapy. These three observations point out the need for a systematic assessment of such developments in a large number of patients so that we can generalize and draw conclusions about specific therapy of greatest benefit to the individual patient.

The importance of comprehensive and detailed short-term and long-term studies of aphasia in cerebrovascular disease is unquestioned. However, every researcher who has tackled a large-scale study is also aware of the limitations of this approach. I would like to discuss these problems briefly and suggest some new lines of investigation which might avoid them.

Among the problems of large-scale studies the difficulties of selective bias; of spotty or redundant examination methods; and of artifacts of sampling produced by selective sampling on reexamination because of death, change of address, hospitalization, or institutionalization are well known. Of even greater importance, however, is the difficulty of classifying patients for analysis. The usual procedure is to use a nosological schema based on medical or on behavioral evidence, in our case on a system of classification for aphasia. The nosological system chosen determines the scope and amount of detail available for analysis. No such schema is likely to produce more than a confirmation or a lack of confirmation for the classification system used by the researcher. In particular we are not able to gain new insights into the usefulness of the nosological schema employed or into the possibility of new types of syndromes of aphasia. This is why large-scale research is often disappointing in its results if one expects more than epidemiological statistics. With all deference to the existing classification of aphasias, it would be useful if we could find a more empirical way of confirming or altering our concepts of the aphasic syndromes, which, to the psychologist at least, appear to have arrived at an almost hopeless impasse. We are not alone with this kind of problem, of course. Classification of the psychiatric disorders faces similar difficulties, although it is gradually inching away from kraepelinian terminology in the wake of several large-scale studies (Guertin and Jenkins, 1956; Lorr, 1961).

If we consider all types of aphasias, not just those of cerebrovascular etiology, we find that some efforts toward more comprehensive studies have already been made. For example, the studies by Schuell, Jenkins, and Carroll (1961), Jones and Wepman (1961), and Howes and Geschwind (1964) have had a primary interest in breaking through the traditional classification and finding new approaches to the analysis of aphasia. In addition, our instruments of investigation are much improved. We have moved from the extremely detailed and sophisticated case study methods of Wernicke (which were usually invented on the spot for a particular patient and rarely repeated with the next one) to comprehensive, standardized testing methods as represented by the batteries of Wepman and Jones (1961), Schuell (1965), Porch (1967), and Spreen and Benton (1968a). Most recently, we have attempted to develop an international, multilingual battery for the assessment of aphasia (Benton, 1969). The use of free speech samples by Howes and Geschwind and by Wepman and Jones has produced an entirely new set of measures of a linguistic and paralinguistic type which can be utilized in the study of aphasic patients.

So far, the fruits of these studies have been meager. Most investigations seem to find support for the traditional classification of aphasias. Schuell's study revived the notion of the unitary nature of all language deficit. Review of these studies shows that most have been designed to confirm or discriminate between types of the traditional classification. The material is sorted into types of deficits defined in advance by the researcher; the data provide confirmation or lack of confirmation for proposed syndromes. Again the sterility of large-scale studies which will yield data only within the framework of a classification chosen at the beginning of the study becomes apparent. No new hypotheses are generated—if indeed there are such new hypotheses in our field.

An exception among these studies in Howes and Geschwind's work with free speech samples (Howes, 1964). Their patients were classified as fast and slow speakers without regard to etiological or conventional classification of aphasia. These behavioral types, i.e., fast and slow speakers, were then compared on a number of other variables, e.g., shape of the log normal distribution of word frequencies and results of supplementary experiments on associations and perceptual thresholds. Only then did the authors review their findings and describe them in relation to standard nomenclature.

Even though this study was limited to a few selected variables of language behavior, it points the way to a more independent approach to aphasia on the basis of behavioral evidence alone, without reference to traditional classification and medical findings. This seems to be the only truly empirical way to reach new definitions of the aphasic syndromes or to confirm the old ones. Geschwind and Howes restricted themselves to two types based on a single variable, i.e., speed of utterances. A multivariable approach, however, is possible with more complex types of analyses, e.g., Lazarsfeld's latent structure analysis (Miller, Eyman, and Dingman, 1961); cluster and factor analysis; and especially Q-type or "inverted" factor analysis (Stephenson, 1953).

A brief description of the Q factor technique illustrates a multivariable approach. The ordinary array of data for a group of patients is transposed or inverted for Q factor technique in such a way that the analysis examines clusters between persons rather than between tests or symptoms. The result of such an analysis consists of "factors" of persons rather than of tests or symptom complexes. Consequently, the interpretation will suggest that each "cluser" of persons forms a relatively homogeneous and separate entity. If the analysis deals with aphasics, the results may be interpreted in terms of patients with distinctive types of aphasias who can empirically be separated from other patients with other types of aphasias. Only at this point can the investigator return to the medical findings and to standard nomenclature and try to identity the aphasia of each group as one of the well-known aphasic syndromes and determine what medical findings the persons with this aphasia have in common.

I would like to include the results of one of our own studies at this point for illustration, but unfortunately cannot because we are still involved in the rather elaborate work of data preparation. A conventional factor analysis with the test data (Spreen and Benton, 1968b) seems to show three distinctive test factors which can be described as "naming and oral speech," "reading, copying, and understanding speech," and "writing, articulation, repetition, and verbal fluency." The more interesting part of the analysis, the search for clusters of persons, has yet to be completed.

This methodology lends itself to the investigation of a classification such as that provided by Geschwind as well as to the generation of new hypotheses about aphasia. If indeed patients with posterior cerebral artery lesions are found to form a "factor" distinctly different from the factors formed by patients with lesions of other types and locations, if there are indeed aphasic syndromes associated with cerebrovascular lesions but not with other types of lesions, the empirical significance of such findings will add considerable strength to our diagnostic and prognostic interpretation.

My second comment concerns our procedures for assessing behavioral change in the study of aphasia. A general treatment of the subject has been presented by Benton (1967).

Geschwind has called our attention to one specific and promising procedure, the Broadbent technique. As applied by Kimura (1961), a *right* ear dominance for two different speech signals presented simultaneously to the two ears can be found for most right-handed persons. More recently, Kimura (1964, 1967), Shankweiler (1966), and Chaney and Webster (1966) reported a *left* ear superiority under similar conditions for nonspeech stimuli, namely, sonar signals and music. In one of our studies, Spellacy (1969) found that this left ear superiority is most clearly evident for music signals but absent or rather weak for isolated components of music such as rhythm, pitch, or timbre. This suggests tentatively that the ear dominance is more a function of the lateral specialization of the association areas than a result of stronger crossed sensory pathways or of a specialization in the immediate auditory receiving cortex. These are speculations, of course; however, the technique seems likely to provide further insight into the pathways involved in this type of performance, both in the right and left hemisphere, and investigations of patients with cortical lesions of various types and locations may be useful. Related opportunities for further study are probably available in the detailed study of sound localization.

My final comment concerns Geschwind's classification of pure alexia without agraphia as a result of lesions involving both the left calcerine cortex and the splenium of the corpus callosum. This type of lesion was also described by Carl Freund (1888) and linked with a different group of symptoms which Freund called "optic aphasia," i.e., a selective impairment of visual naming. About 20 additional cases were reported in the literature until 1900. Most of these patients also suffered from alexia, some with and some without agraphia. Two new cases were reported recently (Spreen, Benton, and Van Allen, 1966) in a study of selective naming disturbance in 20 anomic patients. One of these patients with predominantly visual anomia had alexia and agraphia; the other could read and write well.

Benson and Geschwind (1969) have described the syndrome and the pathology of pure alexia without agraphia in detail, but make no mention of the possibility of a selective naming disturbance as part of this syndrome. A rereading of the earlier literature and a review of our own case material in respect to the presence of alexia and agraphia as well as to type of pathology found the picture to be confusing. For example, our patient who could read and write suffered from a cerebrovascular lesion of undetermined location; our patient with alexia and agraphia suffered from a malignancy deep in the posterior parietal region. The case reports in the older literature on "visual anomia" encompass even more diverse pathology, such as malignancy in the posterior parietal area including the supramarginal gyrus, cerebral abscess after otitis, and stroke. The presence or absence of alexia and agraphia does not appear to be consistently related to type of pathology as far as one can learn from these reports.

This apparent lack of relation between pathology and language disability raises the question whether "visual anomia" may be a common symptom of the "deconnection" type of pathology proposed by Geschwind for alexia without agraphia and, since this seems likely, whether such lesions are indeed primarily produced by cerebrovascular disease.

Again, examination of a series of patients would offer the best prospect of an answer. If this is a special syndrome produced by lesions within the distribution of the posterior cerebral artery, such a picture should emerge more clearly in a large-scale study of the type proposed earlier.

PRESENTATION 7

Frederic L. Darley

The emphasis in the preceding presentations has been on aphasia as a major consequence of cerebrovascular disease with regard to communicative function. To complete the picture, let us remind ourselves that there are several other possible consequences, as Geschwind himself has indicated in some of his writings.

First, patients may have an impairment of motor speech function, i.e., dysarthria, resulting from paralysis, weakness, or incoordination of the speech apparatus. Several patterns of dysarthria can be differentiated, their distinctive features being related to the site of the motor system impairment.

Second, patients may have an articulation difficulty which cannot be attributed to loss of motor power but must be interpreted as difficulty in the programming of speech movements. These patients with what we consider to be apraxia of speech display a speaking performance which is disproportionately poorer than other modality performances in language. They display prominent phonemic errors which are inconsistent, effortful, off-target approximations of the sounds they wish to produce. Their errors are highly variable and are seldom simplifications of the phonemes they wish to produce, in contrast to the dysarthric patients, whose errors tend to be consistent and are usually simplifications. The apractic patients display a marked discrepancy between automatic-reactive speech and volitional-propositional speech. They are usually aware of the errors they make but are often unable to prevent or correct them. In an effort to compensate, the patients present various prosodic changes including slowing of rate, even spacing of words and syllables, and equalization of stress.

Third, patients who are confused display patterns of language disturbance somewhat different from those displayed by aphasic patients. Confused patients characteristically make good responses to specific questions and structured situations, but their responses are poorer to open-ended, less structured questions and situations. Sometimes their responses to such questions are bizarre and irrelevant; sometimes they represent confabulation. Typically the confused patient is not aware of the inappropriateness of his response. His responses are not characterized by word-finding difficulty, phonemic errors, syntactic errors, or disturbed prosody in speech. An associated problem often noted is disorientation in space and time.

Finally, patients with diffuse cerebral disease who display generalized intellectual impairment also demonstrate language impairment which may resemble aphasia: at least mild across-the-board language difficulty; mild auditory retention difficulty; and slowness, vagueness, and unsureness of response. Their attention wanders and they forget what they were doing or talking about or how they were supposed to respond. They express feelings of inadequacy and bewilderment without being aware of specific errors they have made. They display increased difficulty on more abstract tasks. They may or may not be disoriented. But such patients typically do not display syntactic errors; difficulty in recognizing, matching, or naming words, pictures, and objects; bizarre vocabulary; phonetic errors; or confabulation.

It is obvious, then, that when a person administers what is called a "test for aphasia," the errors the patient makes cannot automatically be considered aphasic errors. The nature of the errors, the relative intactness of the various modalities of language, the comparative efficiency of language versus nonlanguage functions, and the associated affective behavior must all be considered in drawing conclusions about the nature of the patient's communication problem.

SECTION III

Language Rehabilitation

PRESENTATION 8

Frederic L. Darley

It is somewhat presumptuous to undertake to review the field of language rehabilitation in aphasia. One is limited largely to published materials, which at best poorly reflect what the practitioners of the art and science of language rehabilitation actually do. Published materials are dated; and if the writer of them had an opportunity, he would update them and doubtless change the concepts or at least their implementing details. The reviewer cannot possibly explain all that enters into an implementation of a therapeutic approach; he cannot describe all the materials or the sequencing of them or the mode of reinforcement of responses or other myriad details that flesh out the skeleton of a therapeutic program. Even though he tries hard, the reviewer is less than omniscient and is bound to overlook important contributions that merit comment. Nevertheless, let us proceed.

EFFECT OF LANGUAGE REHABILITATION

It seems useful first, before talking about various approaches to language rehabilitation, to consider whether data available indicate that language rehabilitation programs are efficacious. Data are not abundant, and the numbers of cases upon which the data are based are relatively few.

Butfield and Zangwill (1946) report on the treatment of 63 patients with aphasia of varied etiology; they indicate that the speech of one-half the patients who began rehabilitation less than 6 months after onset of the disorder, and of nearly one-third of those who began rehabilitation more than 6 months after onset, "was judged to be much improved after re-education." The majority of these patients were young adults. Of the total group, 46 per cent were "much improved," 31 per cent were "improved," the remaining 23 per cent were "unimproved." Their judgments were based on oral speech performance alone. Of their 19 cases of vascular origin, 40 per cent of those treated less than 6 months after onset, and 22 per cent of those treated after more than 6 months, were "much improved."

Wepman (1951) studied 68 young soldiers with largely traumatic head injuries in Army hospitals during World War II, none of whom received language rehabilitation until 6 months after the onset of their problem. Using the Butfield and Zangwill type of rating scale, Wepman reports that 51 per cent of his patients following treatment were much improved and 35 per cent were improved, the remaining 14 per cent being unimproved. Testing of these soldiers led Wepman to believe that as a group they had lost approximately six school grades of achievement in reading, writing, spelling, and arithmetic. Language rehabilitation led to a mean gain of better than five school grades, the greatest gain being made in reading, followed by arithmetic, writing, and spelling. Speech improvement amounted to two steps on a 5-point scale, the mean scale value for the group being 1.8 before training and 3.9 after training, 5.0 on this scale representing normal performance. The mean grade level after training was more than one grade better in those whose training began in the first year than it was in those who began after a whole year had elapsed since onset of the problem.

Marks, Taylor, and Rusk (1957) report on the effects of language therapy on 324 patients, 94 per cent of whom had aphasia of non-traumatic etiology and 64 per cent of whom were over 50 years of age. A 4-point rating scale was used, with the following distribution of results: excellent, 6.9 per cent; good, 22 per cent; fair, 21.4 per cent; and poor, 49.7 per cent.

Godfrey and Douglass (1959) report on a group rehabilitation program with 38 patients where the bulk of the language stimulation was carried on by occupational therapists. They report that progress was good in 37 per cent of the patients and fair in 42 per cent of the patients.

Schuell, Jenkins, and Jiménez-Pabon (1964) present information on 155 patients at the Minneapolis Veterans Administration Hospital. They give no data comparable to those mentioned but do report the percentages of patients who returned to gainful employment in each of Schuell's five classifications. One concludes that a substantial number of patients were helped substantially by the rehabilitation program.

Intermittently in the literature one encounters reference to a study by Luria from which people have drawn conclusions about the normal expectation with regard to spontaneous recovery in aphasic patients. The source is an unpublished manuscript reporting an investigation of 394 brain-injured patients in Moscow. These were largely young patients with traumatically incurred aphasias. Luria reports that 6 months after the onset of the problem only 43 per cent showed "residual signs" requiring reeducation or psychotherapy. The implication is that the other 57 per cent recovered spontaneously within the first 6 months. One might suppose that spontaneous recovery rates would be lower for patients with aphasia of vascular etiology; definitive research on differential spontaneous recovery rates of patients with aphasias of diverse etiology remains to be done. Nevertheless, Godfrey and Douglass (1959) take Luria's figure of 57 per cent and declare it comparable to the "most improved" categories in the studies reported above, the "improved" and other categories by definition being composed of patients who still have progress to make. They say:

> Clearly there is an imperative need for large-scale investigations to provide further data concerning spontaneous recovery rates, but meantime, on the basis of the only data available, any forms of therapy would have to demonstrate considerably more improvement than 40 to 50 per cent, in order to be considered as making significant contribution if the spontaneous recovery rate is 57 per cent. In fact, on the evidence available, there appears to be an inverse relationship between recovery from aphasia and formalized re-education language attempts!

Vignolo (1965) reports on a group of 69 aphasic patients, 42 of whom received language rehabilitation and 27 of whom did not. Briefly, his general conclusion is that the scores for the two groups based upon a scaling of their response to certain language tests indicates no significant difference. But he takes a longer look and says:

> It is also possible that our definition of re-education is too broad and includes patients who are not actually re-educated long enough. If we take only subjects re-educated for more than six months and compare their evolution with that of patients re-educated for less than six months, we find that frequency of improvement is significantly greater in the first group. This holds true also when the two groups are balanced in terms of time from onset and age. . . . Re-education has a specific effect provided that it lasts more than six months. Its influence seems decisive in patients examined for the first time in the period between two and six months from onset.

These data are not overwhelmingly persuasive. I believe that they do tell us, however, that when a systematic program of language rehabilitation is instituted for patients in whom the bulk of improvement attributable to spontaneous recovery has already taken place, i.e., where at least 6 months have elapsed since onset of the problem, and where the rehabilitation program is extended over a period of several months, measurable gains in language achievement can be attributed to the rehabilitation program.

BASIC THERAPEUTIC APPROACHES

Now I would like to discuss approaches to aphasia rehabilitation. There are many ways to classify treatment programs in aphasia, but we will consider two main divisions. The first may be labeled a "stimulation" approach; the goal of therapy is conceived to be the stimulation of the patient to produce the cortical integrations necessary for language, not to educate or reeducate him, not to convey specific new learning or new vocabulary. The second may be called the "programmed instruction" approach; it views language rehabilitation as an educative process and applies in a rigorous way operant conditioning methods drawn from learning theory and principles drawn from psycholinguistic analysis to guide the content and order of presentation of the linguistic elements taught.

STIMULATION APPROACH

Let us first take up the stimulation method. Wepman (1953) has summarized the thinking that underlies this method in his article. He posits three parameters along which all aphasic patients may be placed: stimulation, facilitation, and motivation. Viewing the diverse procedures used by many therapists, all claiming patient gains as a result, he concludes that "what is being done with the aphasic patient in each treatment center is a stimulation process rather than an educative one. . . . All therapists, regardless of their particular approach, are doing what might be called 'stimulation therapy!' " The stimulation provided serves to "reduce the impedance against function by its stimulation effect." He calls *facilitation* a bimodal concept. "It is first the consequence of stimulation, that factor which assists the nonintegrated cortical structure to function in a more integrated manner. At the same time it is a physiological lowering of the impedance against organized cortical action." He goes on to say:

> A mere stimulation of a neural system which is physiologically capable of functioning is not enough, for it is evident clinically that a psychological state of readiness must also exist before maximal learning of the formation of new, operative, neural integrations is possible. . . . Motivation, as the third link in our conceptual chain, indicates the level of goal-directed behavior possessed by the patient. . . . The motivation of the aphasic patient like the motives that move all others must be understood before we can hope to achieve reasonable success in therapy.

Wepman summarizes his concept as follows:

> Stimulation, as used here, means any and every kind of outside, external persuasion, used by those in the patient's environment to provide the individual with stimuli to which he may react. Therapy is organized, goal-directed stimulation, based upon a recognition of the patient's needs, his drives, his motivation. As stimulation is provided at a time when the organism is capable of response it tends to facilitate neural integrations. If the direction of the stimulation at the proper time is in keeping with the patient's psychological state of readiness, if the stimulation is within the modality of language which meets the patient's needs, if the stimulation provides the end reward of realizable and recognizable goals in achievement, then success in therapy is more likely to follow.

We see many ways of implementing this stimulation approach to aphasia rehabilitation. Some are extremely diffuse, simply requiring that everybody around the patient talk to him as much as possible so that he has a great deal of language to react to; the patient may be encouraged to converse with his friends and family, watch TV, listen to the radio, and read out loud. With other practitioners, the method takes a kind of socialization or group psychotherapy approach, aphasic patients meeting together to do pleasant things and interact verbally as much as possible or perhaps meeting together for outpouring of such feelings as they can verbalize, thus coming to feel less isolated, more accepted, less dependent (Blackman, 1950; Aronson, Shatin, and Cook, 1956).

But in most clinics the stimulation method is applied in a more specific way. Wepman describes his use of it in his Army general hospital rehabilitation program (1947, 1951). In the primary stage of recovery he has the nurses and others around the patient talk with him, emphasizing the use of naming words in preference to other parts of speech. He wants them to stimulate the patient and get him using a few words deliberately, confident that soon he will be adding other words by himself.

> All training for aphasia is based upon the fact that it is not the achievement of new learning but rather the integrations necessary for the patient to use his old learning. This is very fortunate indeed for if every sound and every word had to be relearned, recovery for even the best of patients would be an almost endless word-relearning problem and would be even more time consuming than is the integrative learning process. (Wepman, 1951, p. 159)

Wepman encourages the clinician in later stages of recovery to work with the patient on learning more names of things:

> It is often better to select a few common objects and name them several times as they are indicated, not urging the patient to respond in any way.

The series of names is repeated several times. . . . If the patient succeeds in saying anything, one should smile and agree with him, not expecting accuracy of enunciation or completeness of expression. . . . One should continue by picking up the next object and repeating the same process, rewarding every effort and giving the patient all the time he needs to try, whether he succeeds or not. . . . If no success can be obtained by word repetition in this way, adding written clues may be tried. If necessary, one may accompany each showing of the object with an appropriate use of it, showing the patient that the water is for drinking, the book for reading, the pencil for writing, the pipe for smoking, etc.

Wepman suggests that the clinician then go on to hook up verbs with the nouns taught, later to use adjectives and then adverbs, and he warns:

One should not be concerned about the little grammatical words—the prepositions, articles, conjunctions, etc. . . . A typical procedure is to begin with the one-word sentence—the name or noun—following this with the pronouns, especially personal pronouns. After the patient indicates his ability to use a fair number of nouns one should shift to the two-word sentence, the noun plus verb. . . . Simple action verbs that can be demonstrated are best, for example, pencil write, water drink, book read, ball throw, food eat, and others at this level. (Wepman, 1951, p. 180)

Wepman suggests going on in the fairly early stages of training to reading activity, encouraging simple word recognition by having the patient pick words out of the headlines of newspapers, copying words that he knows, reading them aloud, and using them. He suggests the use of all kinds of practice books in reading and writing. He makes use of retired school teachers who have mastered techniques of teaching these skills to children.

The following quotation illustrates some of Wepman's principles of stimulation:

First, use every possible clue and cue. Second, be patient and accepting of every effort. Third, do not stay too long in any one session on the word-finding effort. Fourth, use every person that comes in contact with the patient to assist in the naming process. Fifth, do not urge the use of names on the part of the patient; teach by example. Sixth, imitation of the therapist's use of a name does not appear to be helpful; therefore the therapist should discourage parrot-like repetition. Seventh, give the patient every opportunity to use the name before applying the word. Eighth, stay at the word level if possible. . . . (Wepman, 1951, pp. 239–240)

The usual course of treatment of these patients is to attempt to stimulate them in constantly changing ways. . . .

Successful reduction of aphasic language disturbances is dependent upon a multitude of factors, among which are early diagnosis and referral; careful analysis of the retained and disturbed language functions; proper evaluation of the nonlanguage behavior characteristics; insight into the basic personality of the patient; persistence and patience on the part of the therapist; and cooperation of all of the possible human elements in the patient's immediate environment. (Wepman, 1951, p. 247)

Of course, Wepman says much more. He presents specific suggestions for reducing receptive difficulties of all kinds, teaching the patient to recognize forms, numbers, letters, and words, and to discriminate sizes, colors, and musical notes. He suggests different techniques for direct therapy in expressive aphasia, going back to sounds if necessary, then to words; he advises how to work at writing, how to reteach the use of numbers, etc. By a variety of materials presented in a variety of ways and engaging the patient in a variety of activities, the clinician bombards him, stimulates him, and thus presumably fosters cortical reintegration.

This approach has been updated and further developed by Schuell, Jenkins, and Jiménez-Pabon (1964). In developing her conceptual framework for aphasia, Schuell has a good bit to say about what psycholinguistics can teach us. The conclusions she arrives at are somewhat different from those arrived at by those who advise the programmed instruction approach. Although she recognizes the importance of language structure, she does not teach language structure; she comments:

There is a relatively high correlation between retrieval of words and retrieval of rules at various levels of severity of aphasia. As available vocabulary increases, the beginnings of structure appear. The percentage of well structured responses increases slowly but steadily, although impairment of vocabulary as well as impairment of structural usage continues to be evident.

Schuell defines aphasia as "a general language deficit [see also Schuell and Jenkins, 1959] that crosses all language modalities and may or may not be complicated by other sequelae of brain damage." She continues:

We think the language deficit itself is characterized by reduction of available vocabulary, impaired verbal retention span, and impaired perception and production of messages, perhaps secondary to impairment of the first two dimensions. . . . The evidence for a general reduction of language in aphasia seems clear. All aphasic patients show some impairment of vocabulary and of verbal retention span, with a proportionate amount of difficulty in formulating and responding to messages at some level of complexity. The observed language impairment is not modality specific, and there is an impressive kind of regularity about it. . . . In our model, the language system is an acquired thalamo-cortical organization that functions in the integration and execution of plans involving communication. It receives a flow of processed information from the interacting auditory, sensorimotor, and visual systems, and returns a portion of its output to each subsidiary system for feedback control. Activity in the language system results in storage, indexing, and retrieval of the elements and rules of learned linguistic code, as well as in processing incoming and outgoing messages. . . . We think that aphasia is characterized by impaired retrieval of a learned code, and that this impairment is reflected in all language modalities. Involvement of specific associated sensory systems results in additional impairment, produces identifiable patterns of aphasic deficit, and makes differential diagnosis possible.

Based upon these conceptions, Schuell states:

In our opinion the clinician's role is not that of a teacher. He has nothing to do with teaching the adult aphasic to talk, to read, or to write. He does not teach the patient sounds or words or rules for combining words. Rather he tries to communicate with the patient and stimulate disrupted processes to function maximally.

Schuell then presents a series of seven basic principles of treatment:

1. It would seem that sensory stimulation is the only method we have for making complex events happen in the brain. All the evidence suggests that auditory stimulation is crucial in control of language processes. However, since feedback from more than one sensory modality may contribute to behavior, there is no reason for using this mode exclusively. This suggests that the first principle of treatment for aphasia should be the use of intensive auditory stimulation, although not necessarily stimulation through auditory channels alone. . . . In aphasia, combined auditory and visual stimulation is effective in eliciting language on progressive levels of complexity. It should be continued until the patient can respond to each modality alone on any given level. Skills become functional if this procedure is followed.

2. [The second principle is] that of the adequate stimulus. In other words, we must insure that the stimuli that we use get into the brain. [This involves such precautions as not talking too fast, using meaningful patterns of stimuli rather than nonmeaningful ones, using high-frequency rather than low-frequency words, controlling the length of stimulus, sometimes increasing the loudness of an auditory signal to an optimal level, and manipulating the duration of an auditory stimulus, as in talking more slowly.]

3. [The third principle] involves the use of repetitive sensory stimulation. Over and over, aphasic patients who looked perplexed and bewildered when a word, for example, was spoken once, showed instantaneous recognition when they heard it the fourth or fifth time. . . . The patient who could name five or six out of 20 pictures after 24 hours

when he had received 10 successive auditory stimulations for each word was able to recall from 15 to 20 words the next day, when he received 20 successive stimulations on each word. Someone who has not seen this process in operation may well believe 20 successive repetitions of a single word to involve unbearable monotony, but this is not true.

4. The fourth principle for intensive controlled auditory stimulation is that each stimulus presented should elicit a response. . . . When a patient listens and makes an appropriate response, a whole cycle of activity is set in motion. This cycle involves discrimination, selection, integration, and facilitation of ensuing responses.

5. The fifth principle . . . is that the clinician should elicit, not force, responses. [Techniques vary in their efficiency in eliciting responses; the clinician uses them to enable the patient to respond successfully at each level of recovery.]

6. The clinician should in general stimulate rather than correct. The idea is that defective responses drop out as language functions increase. . . . Clinical time should be spent in stimulation and in eliciting language, not in forcing patients to struggle for responses or in correcting erroneous ones.

7. It is sound procedure to use one language modality to facilitate another throughout the course of treatment. Spelling words aloud helps the patient to write them, hear them, and recall them. Writing sentences to dictation helps him to hear and retain longer language sequences. Reading aloud in unison with the clinician reactivates language patterns, and facilitates speech and reading. (Schuell, Jenkins and Jiminéz-Pabon, 1944, pp. 338–342)

All this, Schuell warns, demands individual work:

> Adult aphasics have only one thing in common, which is a disturbance of communication processes. They present a wide range of individual differences in such significant dimensions as age, intelligence, education, occupation, family background, general interests, physiological and neurological conditions, mental status, and nature and severity of aphasia, as well as other variables. . . . For these reasons, we are unable to have confidence in group therapy as a basic method of treatment for aphasia.

Wepman and Van Pelt (1955) hold a similar view, although they can see that patients who have an apraxia of speech ("motor aphasia") might well work together on the same kinds of problems, being more homogeneous with regard to their problems than are truly linguistically disturbed, i.e., aphasic, patients (Corbin, 1951). Other clinicians have advocated and testified to the usefulness of group therapy for aphasia (Sheehan, 1946; Bloom, 1962).

Similar treatment rationales have been presented by Agranowitz and McKeown (1964), Longerich and Bordeaux (1954), and many others. In his study of the evolution of aphasia with and without language rehabilitation, Vignolo (1965, p. 352–3) summarizes the rehabilitation principles that he and his group have followed; they sound very similar to those mentioned above:

> Therapeutic exercises are viewed as an S-R situation in which the therapist is expected to elicit and consolidate a language response by giving stimuli and reinforcements. The following general rules are kept in mind:
>
> 1. Responses should be as "physiological," i.e., usable in real communication, as possible. In eliciting responses, facilitation is looked for along the lines of the Jacksonian automatic-voluntary dissociation. First an automatic way to elicit a correct response is found, and the response is then tentatively elicited in more and more voluntary ways. Sometimes the patient may be taught to employ the facilitation intentionally as a compensatory round-about way to get to a correct response by himself. However, the habit of using such artificial round-about ways is not encouraged if it is felt that the subject will be able eventually to give physiological verbal responses, i.e., responses which are both highly intentional and highly automatic.
>
> 2. Stimuli and responses involve the lexical and grammatico-syntactic levels of language from the very beginning of therapy. Comprehension and expression of entire and meaningful words and sentences are stressed. Among exercises rehearsing specifically the phonemic level, only those requesting the discrimination and utterance of phonemes within meaningful words and sentences are banned unless anarthria, agraphia or alexia are so complete as to require a rebuilding of the phonemic code itself. This is commonly the case with anarthria, where articulatory and oral apraxic disorders make it necessary to start teaching the articulation movements per se. Such atomistic exercises are abandoned as soon as possible.
>
> 3. The receptive and expressive aspects are both trained together, unless expression is far worse than comprehension (as in severe anarthria). Oral and written language are also drilled together, unless the patient has a global aphasia, in which case reading and writing may be included at the beginning of therapy only if they facilitate the use of oral language.
>
> 4. Finally, emphasis is placed on appropriate use and dosage of reinforcement. Since most exercises may be used for different purposes, reinforcement should vary accordingly and consistently. Right responses are always given a positive reinforcement; wrong ones are regularly given negative reinforcement only in patients with impaired control of speech, while in patients with expressive reduction and blocking they are sometimes better overlooked.

Practically all writers suggest that right responses should always be given positive reinforcement and wrong ones not given negative reinforcement. Stoicheff (1960) presents data showing that responses of patients can vary significantly depending upon the type of instructions they are given and the attitudes that characterize the therapy situation. She shows that patients subjected to a discouraging condition do significantly more poorly at word reading and picture naming than patients who are systematically encouraged and informed of correct performance.

The second main approach to be discussed shortly has drawn heavily from psycholinguistic principles. Before we go on to talk about that approach, the fact should be mentioned that psycholinguistic theory has had considerable impact upon practitioners of the stimulation approach. Scargill (1954) rather early pointed out the implications of linguistics for aphasia therapy in choice of the content of therapy, the use of linguistic signaling devices in facilitating responses, and the importance of working on structural patterns. Schuell, Wepman, Vignolo, and others reflect this importantly in their writings. An interesting example of a specific application of linguistic theory in this method is presented by Beyn and Shokhor-Trotskaya (1966). These Russian practitioners subscribe to the general stimulation approach, for they refer to "the direct method of disinhibiting and stimulating the temporarily inhibited cortical speech functions. This method consists of 'exercising' the disturbed aspects of speech. It yields an appreciable rehabilitative effect and contributes mainly to the elimination of diaschisic phenomena. The direct method of exercising includes: auditory speech stimulation, the use of automatized speech combinations, general activation of the patient's psychic tone, and creation of a 'set' which makes the patient believe in the possibility of rehabilitation."

But within this general framework they set out to try to "prevent the appearance of some of the speech defects of aphasic patients which up to now seemed to be inevitable," specifically the "telegraphic style" of responses, by the introduction of predicative verbal forms before agrammatism becomes manifest. They point out that in the usual practice of language rehabilitation prime importance has been attached to the mastery of object naming, as we saw in Wepman's work and as is illustrated in the materials developed by Taylor and Marks (1959) used so generally around the country, consisting of 100 pictures of objects and accompanying printed words.

The Russians try to lay the foundation for the future development of a normal grammatical system in the patient's speech even when speech is still absent by avoiding the teaching of nominative words and selecting at first only those simplest possible words which can function as a whole sentence—words like "oh," "no," "there," "here," "give," and "take." "The lexical composition of the 'sentences' used in our work with the patients gradually becomes complicated by means of pronouns and adverbs, as well as auxiliary and modal verbs (shall, will, can)." In a second phase they teach expressions such as "give to drink"; "I want"; "I want to eat, sleep, walk"; "I shall eat"; "good"; "bad"; "now"; "tomorrow"; "today"; "yesterday"; "thanks"; "hello." Only when words began to appear spontaneously in a patient's speech are names of objects introduced into it. But these are always used not in the nominative case but in the five Russian oblique cases in which terminations of the nouns change. Expressions are used such as "give me a drink;" "give me the pillow, the coat"; "I am going for a walk"; "I am going to the garden"; "I am reading a book"; "I am writing a letter." Thus when nouns are introduced, they involve morphological changes.

These authors report on work with 25 patients using this method, all patients having an aphasia resulting from cerebrovascular disease. They state: "The results of the rehabilitation of active speech varied; but the most important fact is that telegraphic style, which is *inevitable* with other methods of rehabilitation, did not emerge in any of our patients."

PROGRAMMED INSTRUCTION APPROACH

For some time aphasiologists have been interested in studying the learning behavior of aphasic patients and relating what they have observed to general learning theory. Scattered reports have appeared concerning the application of principles of programmed instruction to the treatment of aphasia, such as those of Tikofsky and Reynolds (1962, 1963), Greenberg (1963), Filby and Edwards (1963), Filby, Edwards, and Seacat (1963), and Rosenberg (1965).

A recent investigation by Carson, Carson, and Tikofsky (1968) demonstrates that although aphasics show limited retention and transfer of learning in general, virtually all 64 subjects studied improved with practice in a specific stimulus-response situation. Although indefinitely long retention was not examined, it is clear that aphasic patients learned some specific skills and retained them over relatively long periods without practice. A considerable area for research is suggested: the relation of nonverbal learning by aphasic subjects to their reacquisition of language, the problems of testing for progress in therapy, the fostering of carry-over of one type of acquired skill to another, and relevance of such learning variables as absolute levels of performance and rates of acquisition.

To our knowledge the first comprehensive program of language rehabilitation for aphasic patients using programmed instruction was developed by Martha Taylor Sarno and her associates at the Institute of Physical Medicine and Rehabilitation, New York University Medical Center. I will borrow from her descriptions of the approach (Sarno, 1964).

The task of the aphasia therapist is a teaching task. [A theoretical framework for language learning can be derived from psycholinguistics, particularly structural linguistics, which] can be called the mathematics of language. . . . The linguist recognizes that the structures of the language can be viewed and analyzed systematically and mathematically, whereas the meanings of words cannot. The unlimited number of variable meanings attached to words cannot be systematically sorted out. . . . The learning of language, in the linguists' view, is not a magical and mysterious process without underlying rationale. It is primarily dependent upon the pattern practice of fundamental structures of the language. These sentence patterns have been identified and analyzed and follow a logical sequence, according to a syntactical order of difficulty. In order for a language to be "learned," an individual must have automatic control of the structures of the language. This is accomplished through the imitation and repetition of the language. . . . To facilitate the establishment of language habits, the linguist suggests that in the process of pattern practice (1) utterances must be short. Patterns should be built only on those structures in vocabulary already learned. (2) Vocabulary should be selected on the basis of frequency of occurrence and only one item at a time should be taught. (3) The immediate reinforcement of a correct response is imperative. (4) Different linguistic features should not be mixed until the response of the individual features of the material to be taught has become automatic.

We see, then, that this approach departs from the traditional emphasis upon vocabulary and concentrates attention instead upon basic structural patterns of language. Sarno alludes to the work of Goodglass and his co-workers (1953, 1960); one of their findings is that the plural form of words is more likely to be retained by aphasic patients than the possessive, despite the fact that these may be identical in their phonemic content; for example, the word *bills* and the possessive *Bill's book*. While these two words are phonemically identical, the operation they perform is different and hence lends each a different place in the hierarchy of difficulty.

Making reference to the work of Skinner (1954, 1957, 1958, 1961), Sarno has drawn upon certain principles of behavioral psychology with special reference to the area of programmed learning. She says:

The field reflects the principle that the conditions for learning can be so arranged that an individual's responses are under the control of the program. In applying this to aphasia treatment, the implication is that the control of the patient's response is in the hands of the therapist and that by properly arranging stimuli, a series of successful responses can be assured, reinforced, and hopefully incorporated in the patient's repertoire of responses. The following characteristics differentiate programmed instruction from other types of teaching. (1) A set of specifications of the instructional goals (terminal behavior) is detailed. (2) The material of instruction is organized into such a carefully designed sequence of small steps that each step is made easier, by virtue of the material previously mastered. In practice, it is found that the optimal step size is usually much smaller than one might think. (3) The learner must be properly reinforced by confirmation of correct responses. . . . (4) The learner must actively participate in the learning process. . . .

The rationales for programmed instruction refer in part to "operant conditioning." Any response that can be rewarded, and which as a result tends to occur more frequently, is an operant. . . . If we desire to change behavior, one way to do it is to wait for the desired response to occur, then reinforce it. But an instructor who follows principles of programmed instruction believes that behavior can be shaped.

Sarno summarizes the approach as follows: "Decide what responses you want to teach; arrange matters so that these responses occur as frequently as possible—with emphasis on success rather than error; reinforce the successful responses."

The N.Y.U.-Bellevue group has developed a comprehensive array of programmed instruction designed to help patients with global or severe aphasia who have not responded to the stimulation approach. Since these subjects are nonverbal, the first programs set out to teach processes considered prerequisite to verbal learning, including imitation of body and then oral movements, visual recognition built around six words (pen, book, one, two, red, and blue), and prewriting (involving tracing, copying, and filling in of geometric forms and names). The first part of the visual recognition program, for example, includes more than 230 steps designed to reach the terminal behavior of matching and selecting objects and picture units with two color and two size variations. The criteria for choice of the six lexical units are (1) ease of phonemic elements; (2) monosyllabic words; (3) size of objects, permitting ease of presentation on a table top; (4) regularity of article required by noun; (5) regularity of grammatical operations; (6) functional useful vocabulary; (7) ease of combining these later into structures without grammatical compromises; (8) ease of visualization of items; (9) facilitation for teaching singular and plural usage in structures later; and (10) high frequency of occurrence in spoken language. Sarno says that "the overall plan was to carry the patient through these pre-verbal programs, then on to programs designed to teach the same lexical items in step-by-step arrangements in each modality—reading, writing, auditory comprehension, and oral production. . . . The total number of steps involved in the complete teaching program on this level is better than 5,000. The actual number of teaching sequences (number of individual programs) is about 20."

Sarno is pleased with the results obtained thus far:

The results obtained in this pilot project have been extremely exciting. They have surpassed our most optimistic expectations. Patients who were unable to learn through other teaching techniques have not only mastered all of the pre-verbal skills, but have proceeded to acquire skills on a much higher level in auditory comprehension and oral production. In one of these cases, the patient's verbal impairment was of over one year's duration and considered to be irrevocable.

Certain observations in this particular informal pilot program are of special interest. While the material appears monotonous and repetitious, patients have demonstrated maximum attention to the presentation of programmed materials. They have evidenced a persevering capacity with this method, whereas other methods usually did not hold their attention. The anxiety, so blatantly expressed in many severely impaired aphasic patients, was reduced dramatically. Patients who had numerous catastrophic reactions to other methods, did not exhibit any catastrophic symptoms. Patients with minimal fatigue thresholds tolerated much longer periods of training.

In addition, our experience in programming instruction for aphasic patients in this pilot project has confirmed many of the advantages often cited. Programmed instruction (1) enables patient to work at his own rate of language learning; (2) has built-in measurements of language learning; (3) forces the clinician to work at patient's real level of functioning; (4) has built-in systematic record of responses to act as feedback for programming; (5) forces us to analyze terminal behaviors and approximately design materials and methods for their realization; and (6) forces and facilitates a markedly increased precision in the description of language recovery for charts, progress notes, research, and so forth.

I have only told you of the positive and rewarding aspects of this technique in aphasia rehabilitation. But there are some significant disadvantages. The greatest, perhaps, is that therapists somehow do not like programmed instruction. They continue to believe that the therapist's role in aphasia rehabilitaton should be creative. It should also be noted that the amount of careful planning, analysis, and expense required for the design of the simplest program is extraordinary.

Sarno and Sands (1967) report the following more specific data from their pilot study:

The 25 aphasic subjects studied in the pilot project were all right-handed, right hemiplegic, native speakers of English who had sustained cerebrovascular accidents. All had a premorbid history of normal verbal behavior. Each patient received a half-hour session five times weekly for an average period of 2.6 months. All subjects were severely impaired; each had an overall score of less than 20 per cent on the Functional Communication Profile, indicating an absence of meaningful oral output and marked impairment of auditory comprehension. If a patient failed to achieve the terminal behavior after a two month trial, a comparable program in a different modality or process was administered.

The average length of time spend on a single program was one week, although some patients worked for as long as one month on one program.

The results were as follows:

1. Twenty-one of twenty-five patients achieved at least one of the terminal behaviors in one or more language modalities.

2. More than 25 per cent of the patients significantly reduced their errors in repeated trials of a single program. As much as a 30 per cent error reduction was noted in several cases.

3. Motivation was rated as "increased," "decreased," or "the same" by the therapists responsible for carrying out treatment. Twenty patients demonstrated increased motivation for speech therapy when Programmed Instruction was administered.

4. Patients learned to inhibit extraneous physical movements during programmed treatment sessions and to pay attention to specific stimulus items for longer periods of time than was possible under non-programmed techniques.

5. Subjects who were unable to learn to imitate phonemes under non-programmed techniques learned this task when presented with a programmed method.

6. Patients who were usually unable to inhibit meaningless utterances learned to inhibit this behavior while receiving oral production programs.

7. Subjects who were unable to trace geometric forms learned to trace and copy these forms and, ultimately, to copy entire words.

8. All patients who were given the program designed to teach name writing succeeded in learning this task with few or no errors.

9. A Programmed Instruction method seemed to increase patients' awareness of their own errors, a necessary prerequisite to language learning.

10. Those who received Programmed Instruction appeared to retain material for a longer period of time than those who were taught by non-programmed teaching methods.

EVALUATION OF THERAPEUTIC APPROACHES

Can we evaluate the relative merits of these two main approaches? The rationale presented by Wepman and developed by Schuell for the stimulation approach is compelling. All of us who have used it have seen many patients make measurable progress in response to stimulation. The more carefully organized, graded, and sequenced, in general the better pleased we have been with our results. We have all experienced plenty of failures through the use of this method.

Sarno and her associates have used the programmed instruction approach for a limited number of years but have presented us with some persuasive data about its effectiveness with precisely those patients whom the rest of us have failed with using the stimulation approach.

Both these approaches involve features which, as has been stated, sound terribly repetitious, monotonous, and dull. Yet the advocates of both approaches indicate that with the kinds of patients on whom they have been successful, they have not been experienced as monotonous and dull. In both approaches as patients experience success, they express enthusiasm for rehabilitation activities and can participate actively in them.

The stimulation approach seems to require more art on the part of the therapist, more creativity, more intuition. The programmed instruction approach involves an astonishing initial investment of time and effort but appears to be more rigorous, repeatable, and measurable in its effects. Research has yet to be done which will tell us the relative merits of the two approaches with comparable groups of appropriately selected patients, as well as the limitations of the approaches with certain kinds of patients or in certain kinds of settings or with certain types of language functions.

APRAXIA OF SPEECH

One type of so-called "aphasia" does not belong in the disorder whose treatment we have discussed up to this point. I am speaking of the entity initially called aphemia by Broca and subsequently referred to by such names as Broca's aphasia, motor aphasia, subcortical motor aphasia, anarthria, verbal aphasia, expressive aphasia, apraxia, apractic dysarthria, and phonetic disintegration of speech. More and more of us are coming to call this problem by the name that Liepmann applied to it—apraxia. We are referring to the difficulty the patient has in programming articulatory movements and therefore expressing himself orally, even though he presents no significant weakness or incoordination of the speech mechanism, his comprehension is essentially intact, and he can express himself alternatively in writing.

From the very beginning Broca did not confuse this problem with a generalized language loss. He called the loss of the faculty of articulated language "aphemia," whereas he called impairment of the general faculty of language "verbal amnesia." The distinction has at times seemed almost to have been lost, but then has again been clarified. In his 1951 book Wepman made a distinction between the treatment of apraxia of speech and aphasia. He and Van Pelt later emphasized the distinction (Wepman and Van Pelt, 1955). Agranowitz and McKeown (1964) set forth a completely different kind of treatment for patients with this kind of disorder than for those with a truly linguistic disturbance.

Since the problem of these patients is in the programming of motor acts, what has been called a direct method of therapy usually seems efficacious. One makes use of the mirror in direct confrontation with the patient to show him how sounds are made and to help him make use of all visual, kinesthetic, and tactile cues at his disposal. Whereas drill does not work in aphasia, drill is most effective in apraxia. We start with single sounds and show the patient how to produce a sound in isolation, then putting the sound into syllables, first in the initial position, then in the final, and then building more complicated units such as two-syllable words in which the sound appears at the beginning of both syllables, like "mama," or two-word sequences, such as "my money," where the pattern is repeated. More and more consonant patterns are built; then the patient practices discriminating and differentially producing the patterns he has up to that time been confusing, such as the frequent substitution of *t* for *k* and vice versa.

We know of no study of the efficacy of treatment for apraxic speech. It is our personal experience and that of others that what works with aphasic patients does not work with apraxic patients and vice versa. We have worked effectively with several patients presenting a pure or relatively pure apraxia of speech who have made excellent progress.

ADJUNCTS TO THERAPY

MEDICATION

Only scattered and contradictory reports tell us about the use of drugs as adjuncts to rehabilitation programs for aphasic patients. Reports by Linn and Stein (1946), Linn (1947), Billow (1949), Bergman and Green (1951), and D'Asaro (1955) present equivocal findings concerning the effects of Sodium Amytal on aphasic performance. Smith and Turton (1951) suggest the possible beneficial results of vasodilating drugs on patients whose aphasia is secondary to cerebral arteriosclerosis. We have known of scattered efforts to use mood elevating drugs such as Ritalin, but systematic control studies remain to be reported.

HYPNOSIS

Recognizing that aphasic behavior, though organic at base, presents many functional components, clinicians have wondered whether language function might be improved in hypnotic trance or through posthypnotic suggestion. To our knowledge a single report exists in the literature (Kirkner, Dorcus, and Seacat, 1953) describing the use of hypnosis, not in a bona fide case of aphasia, but rather in a patient with "a complete ideokinetic apraxia of speech which is equivalent to motor aphasia." The usual speech retraining efforts had failed to produce any vocalization on the part of the patient. With the aid of hypnosis, he was induced to vocalize. Following this, oral speech retraining proceded in the traditional way with good result.

Further exploration of the possible adjunctive benefits of both medication and hypnosis are needed. One deterrent to such research in the past has been the absence of sufficiently objective and quantitative procedures for measuring small changes in language behavior. We believe that the need for such a measuring instrument has now been met by the Porch Index of Communicative Ability (Porch, 1967), which provides for the rating on a 16-point scale of each of 10 performances on each of 18 language subtests. Porch's standardization data indicate that the instrument is useful in reliably reflecting even small increments of improvement in language function.

MACHINES

Many clinicians have developed automated techniques of various kinds in an attempt to provide some variety in the clinical situation and also to supplement direct clinical work with patient self-help techniques. Perhaps best known is the Language Master and the sets of stimulus materials developed by Moore and Schuell. The use of a specific language board is described by Keith and Darley (1967). A conference concerning the use of such machines was held at Ohio State University in October 1968.

HOME PROGRAMS

As the number of aphasic patients has increased and a shortage of qualified personnel to deal with them has persisted, many aphasiologists have endeavored to enlist the help of the family in providing language stimulation, though others have deplored the practice and advised against it (Boone, 1967). Perhaps the best known of these home programs was developed by Taylor and Marks (1959). Among other materials specifically designed for this purpose are those of Longerich (1958), Decker (1960), Houchin and DeLano (1964), and Agranowitz and McKeown (1964). Useful informational booklets for lay consumption include those by Longerich (1955), Taylor (1958), Boone (1961), the Kenny Institute (Peterson and Olsen, 1964), and the American Heart Association (1965).

OTHER ASPECTS OF THE IMPACT OF THERAPY

Up to this point, I have not discussed the "psychological" benefits of therapy. We have no empirical studies that clearly define these less tangible consequences of therapy, but the clinician encounters daily evidence that his interaction with the patient yields benefits beyond linguistic parameters.

The aphasic patient has suffered an amputation of his capacity to interact and communicate with his fellow men, sometimes mild, sometimes severe, but nevertheless an amputation. This constitutes a threat not only to his earning capacity but to his identify as an individual and a human being. Even though a relatively bland exterior may mask it, the pervading emotion is essentially panic. Goldstein called it "the catastrophic reaction," and it is always at the threshold. Its imminence varies with the understanding the patient has of the nature of the problem, his expectations regarding its outcome, the acceptance he encounters in those around him, and the degree to which the expectations and demands of those around him serve to help and reassure him or serve to provoke him.

The clinician in therapy continually provides information, insight, encouragement, and optimistic effort; he assuages tendencies to self-criticism and self-punishment, anxiety, and despair. By his supportive, nonprovocative manner and his systematic schedule of language stimulation he conveys to the patient that the problem is understood and can be dealt with constructively. The clinician typically also extends his efforts beyond the patient to the patient's associates so that they, too, will have adequate information and insight about what is going on and do the helpful things for the patient rather than those that provoke, unduly pressure, dishearten, and push him to the brink of the catastrophic reaction.

Patients' testimony constitutes the best documentation of the importance of this aspect of language rehabilitation. We should not dismiss it as nebulous or of only sentimental significance. It is an essential ingredient of the clinical situation and perhaps in some cases the only ingredient that makes a great deal of difference.

CONCLUSION

This, then, is at least one man's view of language rehabilitation. We are doing better than we did when World War II produced many brain-injured servicemen whose plight demanded attention in the form of patched-together programs operated by well-meaning but largely untrained workers from several professions. The sheer number of patients we have seen has taught us a lot about what works and what does not work. Systematic research on these patients has taught us more. Experimental psychology and psycholinguistics have given us new tools and encouraged greater rigor in selection of stimulus materials; selection of contingencies and schedules; and accuracy of observation, measurement, and reporting. The art is giving way to the science of language rehabilitation, but, it is hoped, with the aphasic patient and his needs still occupying stage center.

Schuell and her associates (1964) have said eloquently:

> It is irresponsible to treat a patient without comprehensive information about the problem he presents. But the clinician must also deal directly with a human individual, and often with one upon whom suffering, physical weakness, anxiety, and other sequelae of incapacitating illness have imposed their inexorable indignities and humiliations. This is the hard fact the clinician cannot turn away from if he is to help the patient assimilate traumatic experiences so that healing can occur. In addition the clinician requires a hard core of scientific knowledge, if he is to help the patient more than any kind, well-meaning, but untrained person can. Professional competence is never an absolute achievement but is, rather, something in the nature of a lasting commitment.

PRESENTATION 9

Donald P. Shankweiler

There is little I can add to Darley's informative review of what has been written about language rehabilitation. I can only second his complaint that the conflicting claims are many and the difficulties in resolving them formidable. I think it must be said that there are few hard data to support a belief that speech therapy aids recovery from aphasia. This point has often been misunderstood. The question is whether specific procedures can be shown to influence the outcome of aphasia. Speech therapy has sometimes been considered so broadly as to make impossible scientific scrutiny of its effects. The need for sympathy and psychological support during recovery from catastrophic illness accompanied by sudden loss of function can be taken for granted. While not discounting the supportive, morale-sustaining aspect of their role, I think most speech therapists and speech pathologists view their function as providing diagnosis and treatment of a more specific kind, and in considering the question of the efficacy of speech therapy, I wish to examine the belief that treatment can have a direct influence on the course and extent of adaptation to injury or disease.

Ideally, evaluation of the efficacy of a particular treatment involves the comparison of matched pairs of individuals, one of whom receives the treatment the other does not, but who are otherwise much alike in age, etiology and symptoms of disorder, educational attainments, and time since onset of the illness. In practice it is very difficult to assemble such groups, and to assemble enough different kinds of groups to evaluate the effects of the variables of age, etiology, presenting symptoms duration of symptoms before beginning treatment, duration of treatment, and interactions among these variables is a very large task. Vignolo (1965), in a paper discussed by Darley, states the case well for properly controlled studies for evaluating the effects of therapy. He painstakingly exposes the difficulties, both practical and conceptual, which stand in the way of really definitive studies which would give a clear answer to the question whether therapy X is better than therapy Y, and, in turn, better than no therapy.

It is the nature of speech and language disturbances to change in the course of time following the onset of the injury or disease. We have to evaluate any effect of treatment against the background of change which is part of the recovery process. Vignolo stresses that in order to do this successfully we have to know more than we do about the recovery process, the "spontaneous evolution" of aphasia, and with this point I heartily agree.

Vignolo examined the records of 69 adult patients with aphasia of nontraumatic etiology, and after frankly discussing the unavoidable shortcomings and limitations of the study, addressed himself to three broad questions:

1. Does spontaneous evolution of aphasia occur? Do the characteristics of the disorder tend to change in any particular direction? Do aphasic syndromes generally tend to improve or deteriorate spontaneously?

2. What is the influence of natural factors, such as age, type of aphasia, etc., on the course?

3. Does language rehabilitation influence evolution and, if so, under what conditions? Should therapy be undertaken before or after the period of spontaneous recovery?

In answer to the first question Vignolo concluded that disturbances of oral expression and comprehension in aphasia undergo spontaneous evolution in the direction of recovery of function, but that receptive functions improve more than expressive functions. As to the effect of age, improvement appears to be much less frequent in old people than in young people. The proportion of persons who show significant improvement decreases as the time interval from onset of symptoms to the initial examination increases over a range from 0 to 6 months. As for the effect of therapy itself, the general comparison between patients who received it and those who did not showed no significant difference when the groups were balanced with respect to the other variables mentioned above. Vignolo, because of his thorough appreciation of the complexity of the problem of evaluation, did not, as Darley has pointed out, state this negative result without qualification. He then compared subjects who received therapy for more than 6 months with those who received it for less than 6 months and found the frequency of significant improvement greater in the first group, and he showed that this difference is not an artifact of time of onset or age. His tentative conclusion was, then, that treatment extended over 6 months is of value in aphasia rehabilitation.

A study made by Sands, Sarno, and myself (1969) on an even smaller group bears out many of Vignolo's conclusions. Our group was comparable to Vignolo's in that it included patients with aphasia of nontraumatic etiology. Of all the variables we considered, we found age to be the most important predictor of extent of recovery. We, as Vignolo, found that the average length of treatment for the portion of our group which improved most was considerably longer (15 months) than for that portion which improved least (8 months). I do not think, however, that these figures or Vignolo's can be taken to mean that treatment is more effective if it is continued longer. Patients in our group, and presumably in Vignolo's as well, were in fact retained in therapy only as long as they continued to show measurable gains, so the comparison is not simply between two randomly selected groups of patients arbitrarily assigned to different lengths of treatment.

A question of some importance is, when should therapy begin? To approach this question we considered separately those of our patients whose treatment had begun no later than 2 months after the occurrence of the stroke and those whose treatment had begun after 4 months. As it turned out, the numbers for this comparison were about equal. There was a definite advantage for the early treatment group. The interpretation of this finding is equivocal, however, since, other things being equal, we may expect that the "early" group had still more to gain from spontaneous recovery than the "late" group. Therefore, we cannot necessarily attribute the greater improvement of the early treatment group to therapeutic intervention. Neither can we exclude the possibility that early treatment is advantageous.

My purpose in discussing these studies at some length is less to affirm the findings than to illustrate the variety and complexity of the problems which must be faced if we are to demonstrate the efficacy of treatment for aphasia. Vignolo has pointed out that the complexity of the problem calls for large-scale, long-term, multivariate investigations with elaborate research designs for assessing the interactions among the many variables. I believe such a study is now premature. First, as Vignolo has stressed, the task requires that an objective evaluation of the disorders be made. We have first to identify the salient features of the disorders we wish to treat. An objective system of classification and description is a requirement for designing a rational therapy. We are far from such a system at present. Second, unless understanding of the nature of the disorder has provided a specific rationale for treatment, there will be no therapeutic procedures that are definite enough and stable enough to evaluate. I will discuss each of these points in turn.

Darley and others have commented on the chaotic state of classification in aphasia. We know this problem is not merely a matter of multiple terminologies which could in principle be reconciled and standardized in the interests of communication. Unfortunately, the multiple terminologies and classifications reflect to a large extent a lack of agreement about what the salient facts are. For the most part, the research on which an adequate classificatory system might be based has not been done. I would stress that the needed research is not to be viewed chiefly as a matter of standardizing and quantifying our observations, although these things are important. The task is more difficult than the application of a technology of measurement. We have first to discover the right observations, namely those which lead to a theory of the disorder which accounts for the symptoms, such a theory would generate rather specific proposals for treatment. To demonstrate that these proposals do indeed work would be one kind of evidence for the correctness of the theory. I know of few instances in which an approach to treatment grew out of experimental analysis of the disorder in question. One such instance is the approach to treatment of articulatory disorder in motor aphasia as outlined by Darley, Luria (1963), and others. I will return to discuss the problem of articulatory disorder shortly, but by way of introduction, I would like to mention Luria's views on what speech therapy is about.

In a remarkable little book called *Restoration of Function After Brain Injury*, Luria (1963) develops a rationale for the treatment of a broad range of impairments of perceptual and motor skills and of language and speech following damage to the cerebral hemispheres. The procedures described in the book are largely an outgrowth of the author's war experience and hence are concerned almost exclusively with the effects of traumatic injuries, but the principles he puts forth may also be of interest in rehabilitation of patients with cerebrovascular disease. As is usual with Luria, the documentation of the claims is sketchy, but the ideas themselves are interesting and merit consideration.

Luria argues cogently that there is a good deal more to the recovery process than disinhibition or diaschisis. Because of the irreversible effects of destruction of brain tissue, recovery is less a matter of restoration of a behavior pattern in its original form than a reorganization of the pattern in an altered form. Two types of reorganization are distinguished. First, there is automatic reorganization; some of the examples given are transfer of simple grasping functions from the paretic hand to the sound hand and reorganization of seeing after an injury leaving only part of the visual field intact. The second type of reorganization of function requires the cultivation of deliberate strategies of compensation for a defect. Such compensation does not take place automatically, but rather requires special training. The example is given of restoration of articulated speech in some varieties of motor aphasia. This is a problem of considerable interest both to Darley and to my colleagues and me (Shankweiler and Harris, 1966; Shankweiler, Harris, and Taylor, 1968), and it illustrates an aspect of language rehabilitation in which clear goals for treatment can be stated together with fairly specific guidelines for achieving these goals. This is possible, I would argue, because it is known what kinds of distortions these patients make when they attempt to produce a phoneme string.

Disturbances of articulated speech are a prominent feature in many cases of motor aphasia. Many patients present difficulty in programming articulatory movements as their chief difficulty. In some, it can be demonstrated that comprehension is essentially intact and the patient can express himself well in writing. Darley, Luria, and my colleagues at the Institute of Rehabilitation Medicine in New York all report that a direct approach to this disorder often seems to meet with obvious success. The task described by both Darley and Luria is really to teach the patient the basic elements of articulatory phonetics. What is lost in this disorder, either partially or relatively completely, is the automatic ability to carry out phonemic encoding, an aspect of language which is an acquisition of very early childhood, largely complete by age 3. Many patients can never regain the automatic use of this code, but they can by hard practice and imitation learn to produce and sequence phonemic gestures to produce intelligible, though defective speech. By use of every device he can command, the therapist teaches the patient all the fundamental positions of the articulators required for the pronunciation of a given speech sound. Luria sees in this retraining situation a paradigm for rehabilitation work in other aspects of language, as well as other skills. He characterizes it as the "transfer of the defective operation to the patient's consciousness" by teaching the mastery of normally unrecognized rules.

Luria believes this paradigm has wide applicability. I do not know whether it does, but I think it is true that the rules of language are at present best understood at the level of phonology, and I submit that it is at this level that we may achieve the most in understanding aphasia, if only because scientific techniques are already available from psychology, physiology, and the phonetic sciences for the study of the determinants of speech perception and production.

To summarize, I think there can be no categorical answer to the question whether speech therapy works in aphasia. It depends on the nature of the patient's disorder, whether he is young or old, what kind of lesion he has, how severely affected by the disease are his remaining capacities and motivation, the type of treatment he receives, and many other variables. Large-scale studies to evaluate the efficacy of treatment are premature, because we are not on the whole in agreement about how to assess language function or in a position to be sufficiently explicit about the therapy program. On the other hand, specific treatment programs, which grow out of an analysis of the salient features of a particular disorder, can and should be subjected to scientific study.

PRESENTATION 10

D. Frank Benson

In any discussion of the value of aphasia therapy, one point should be made clear. Aphasic patients vary considerably, and the response to treatment is accordingly variable. It is my opinion, based on observation rather than on statistical studies, that certain types of aphasic disturbances respond better to therapy than others. Specifically, we seem to have our best results with so-called conduction aphasia, quite frequently have good results with Broca's aphasia, and recently have had outstanding improvement in several patients with pure word deafness. The results in therapy depend upon a number of variables—not only the clinical type of aphasia but also the severity of the causative brain disorder and the motivation for therapeutic improvement displayed by the patient. Obviously, the skill and experience of the therapist also plays a significant part.

We are performing a long-term investigation of aphasia therapy at the Boston Veterans Administration Hospital. This is not a comparison of treated and untreated patients, but an investigation of the efficacy of Dexedrine as an adjunct during aphasia therapy. We are actually carrying on this investigation as two separate studies, one using patients who have been aphasic for over 6 months without significant language improvement and the other using patients who have been aphasic for 2 and 3 months. The first group acts as its own control, but both studies are double-blind. All patients are given capsules. One-half receive capsules with Dexedrine and the other half capsules containing an inert placebo. Extensive speech function and psychological testing is performed prior to starting treatment; the patients then enter into or continue aphasia therapy programs appropriate for their specific disorder. They remain in therapy for 3 months and at the end of the therapy period are fully retested. They are retested again 1 month after the medication has been discontinued. From this study we hope to demonstrate the efficacy, if any, of Dexedrine medication during aphasia therapy. Studies modeled on this investigation could be used for other studies of aphasia therapy.

SECTION IV

Psychomotor and Vocational Rehabilitation

PRESENTATION 11

Leonard Diller

Any discussion of such an imposing topic as psychomotor and vocational rehabilitation is beset with a number of difficulties which ought to be acknowledged at the outset:

1. While hemiplegia is treated by many students in the field as a unitary disability with associated handicapping conditions, this is by no means an actual fact. During the acute phase there appear to be distinctive subtypes which may be obscured with the passage of time. Indeed Fisher (1965, 1967; Fisher and Curry, 1965), in describing a number of syndromes, has used the term "pure motor hemiplegia of vascular origin" despite the seeming redundancy, because the term hemiplegia has become practically synonomous with any one-sided stroke.

2. Normative data on sensory and motor capacities are sparse for the age groups usually susceptible to hemiplegia (Welford, 1959; Woodburne, 1967).

3. While some data are available concerning certain complex functional motor skills, we lack adequate neuropsychological information for understanding the mechanisms of complex functional skills or orientation in space (Freedman, 1968).

4. Many specific parameters noted in the course of clinical work are part of the experiences of all sophisticated neurological and physiatric observers. These include motor power, range of motion, spasticity, rigidity, ataxia, pain, sensory changes, and mental confusion, which have been described many times (Treanor and Psaki, 1954; Moskowitz, Bishop, and Shibutani, 1958; Peszczynski and Bruell, 1960; Moskowitz and Porter, 1963; Rusk, 1964; Hastings, 1965).

5. There are very few prospective longitudinal studies of sensory and motor recovery in untreated patients (Twitchell, 1951; Bard and Hirschberg, 1965).

Rather than review all the salient considerations of psychomotor and vocational rehabilitation, I will limit discussion to those areas in which psychology and rehabilitative medicine contribute cooperatively to the improvement of the hemiplegic patient. I will consider the following topics: improving ability in activities of daily living, changing behavior in the clinical situation, changing behavior under laboratory conditions, and vocational problems in hemiplegia.

IMPROVING ABILITY IN ACTIVITIES OF DAILY LIVING

Activities of daily living, or ADL as they are commonly termed in rehabilitation circles, consist of the most common functional motor skills which are part of the normal behavior necessary for an individual to function independently in our society. The functional aspect of these skills is salient. The patient is not taught a motor skill: He is taught to walk, to dress himself, to wash his hands. ADL are correlated with motor acts but are not identical with them. For example, combing the hair and brushing the teeth may be contingent on grasp and release, but they constitute more than grasp and release. Adler and Tal (1965) divided ADL functions into four categories in terms of degrees of independence and then studied their hemiplegic patients in terms of a 4-point scale of motion impairment. On this scale, 1 indicated almost full range of motion and 4 indicated no movement in upper limb, no hip and ankle movements, severe spasticity with contractures. Although the association between these two measures was highly significant in a sample of 293 patients, in only 109 of the 293 cases was there an exact congruence between the 4-point ADL scale and the 4-point motion-impairment scale.

RATIONALE FOR ADL SCALES

While ADL have long been of interest to the clinical worker concerned with improving the lot of his patient, their formalization as a therapeutic objective of treatment or as a scale was slower. For example, modern notions that the scientific study of human movements could be applied to the treatment of diseased states may be seen as far back as the nineteenth century (Kouindjy, 1920; Hirt, 1967), and the well-known muscle test (Beasley, 1961) was devised by Lovett (1916) to deal with an outbreak of poliomyelitis, but ADL as a formal area of rehabilitation which can be measured and used as a base line for admission, evaluation of progress, and discharge from a rehabilitation program did not gain wide acceptance until the 1940's. Today ADL scales are being used not only in this country, but all over the world Broman and Lindberg-Broman, 1965).

The clinical worker typically evaluates the patient on his competence in a number of tasks and records his performance on forms or check lists. The criteria for the selection of tasks have generally involved two considerations: (1) the task must be an important and commonly performed act which is marred by a disabled state due to disease, and (2) the act should be susceptible to modification by exercise, training, devices, or other means which the worker has at hand. Evaluating the competence with which an act is performed poses a problem, since the usual criteria of speed and accuracy utilized in the study of psychomotor skills of normal individuals (Noble, 1968) may be less sensitive and less practical than the criterion of how much assistance the individual needs to complete the act. It is of interest to note that the writer could find no studies using time and accuracy of performance of ADL tasks as criteria of progress in the rehabilitation of hemiplegics.

As a system of evaluation, the ADL scale has one major virtue: The individual tasks have immediate and obvious validity. Unlike other methods of measurement, e.g., intelligence tests or achievement tests, the ADL tasks bear an intuitive rather than a statistical affinity with the criterion. ADL tasks are intrinsically adapted to a criterion of functional daily living. In reviewing the history of ADL scales, we may note three stages: (1) an attempt to develop the scales and demonstrate their usefulness in working with the neurologically impaired (Brown, 1960); (2) an attempt to use the scales to demonstrate the usefulness of rehabilitation (Dinken, 1947; Lee *et al.*, 1958); (3) an attempt to use the scales as a critical indicator of the value of rehabilitation versus other forms of treatment (Benton, Brown, and Rengler, 1951; Gordon *et al.*, 1962; Gordon and Kohn, 1966). With this shift in orientation there is now a tendency to look at ADL scales more critically (Kelman and Willner, 1962), and future studies in this field may be expected to reflect this increased sophistication (Schoening *et al.*, 1965).

Despite these subtle shifts in attitudes toward ADL scales, not all workers in the field would agree to quantifying ADL or dealing with the scales in a standardized way. Brown (1960), in her review of the development of ADL as an important area for treating the disabled, commented that when she was working on her evaluation form more than 2 decades ago, she presented it to Arnold Gesell and his staff, who urged that it be used as a clinical tool rather than a psychometric instrument. The reasons for this point of view are the presumed idiosyncratic nature of patients, their disabilities, their environments, and the staff who diagnose and treat them. While the merits of this point of view cannot be denied, the growing interest in rehabilitation and in chronic disease as a public health problem, has led to a need for standardized instruments to evaluate the effectiveness of programs. For example, there has been recent discussion on the optimum place of treatment for hemiplegic patients. Arguing from data derived from ADL performances, some have advocated programs housed in rehabilitation settings (Covalt, 1952; Rosenblatt, 1961); others have argued for community-based programs which feature therapists carrying out home visits (De Lagi *et al.*, 1962; Ragoff, Cooney, and Kutner, 1964). Some have used ADL scales to evaluate effectiveness of applying rehabilitation procedures to disabled persons living in nursing homes (Kelman and Muller, 1962; Kelman and Willner 1962; Gordon and Kohn, 1966), geriatric wards (Rae, Smith, and Lenzce, 1962), and general medical wards (Adams and McComb, 1953; Carroll, 1962; Feldman *et al.*, 1962). It is clear that without common standardized ways of evaluating functional performance, meaningful discussion of the effectiveness of treatment is foreclosed. Furthermore, a formal standardized scale has the virtue of forcing the worker to make his criteria for selecting items of behavior more explicit. Having to translate a clinical observation into a standard language sharpens the thinking of the translator.

COMPOSITION OF ADL SCALES

There is wide disagreement on the number of domains of activity to be covered by ADL scales. The most common approach is to divide ADL into two basic domains: degree of independence of ambulation and degree of independence in self-care (Andersen, Hanvik, and Brown, 1950; Zarling, 1954; Lee, 1958; Feldman *et al.*, 1962; Gordon *et al.*, 1962; Gordon and Kohn, 1966). The boundaries of these domains are not clear: For example, Feldman *et al.* (1962) include travel as part of locomotion. Various writers have defined domains in different ways: For example, Kelman and Muller (1962) considered ADL to consist of five areas—transfer, toilet, locomotion, feeding, and dressing; Schoening *et al.* (1965) considered six areas—bed activities, transfers, locomotion, dressing, personal hygiene, and feeding; De Lagi *et al.* (1962) evaluated functioning in eight areas; and Carroll (1962) evaluated functioning in twelve areas.

The problem of how many separate areas to include may be considered in terms of the purposes of the study, as Gordon and Kohn (1966) have suggested. For certain heuristic purposes, it may even be desirable to concentrate on a single functional activity, as did the classical study of dressing difficulties in individuals with damage to the right hemisphere (Brain, 1941; Paterson and Zangwill, 1944) which preceded our current interest in hemispheric differences on mental tests by a decade and a half. It is not clear, however, that analysis of a single activity is sufficient to provide specific guidance in clinical work. Schoening and Iverson (1968) suggested that tasks and domains to be included in an ADL scale be chosen with regard to reliability; validity; similarity of activity in strength, coordination, and mobility requirements; and extent of time required by assistive personnel if the patient is not independent. The separate domains of behavior included in a valid profile of ADL functioning easily lend themselves to multivariate analyses, particularly factor analysis.

SCORING OF ADL SCALES

The number of scale points utilized in studies of hemiplegia have ranged from 2 (Lowenthal, Tobis, and Howard, 1959) to 100 (Wylie, 1966). Some writers identify the points on the scales in terms of a clinical judgment (e.g., adequate–inadequate); others in terms of behavior. The problem is to describe an act in terms of the degree of success with which it is executed. The most common standard is to delineate success in terms of the amount of assistance the individual needs to complete the act. This measure, typical of the pragmatic-mindedness of the rehabilitation movement, may be useful for statistical purposes but may obscure more probing analysis. For example, 2 patients may require "moderate" assistance for different reasons or 2 patients may "improve" to the same extent in their requirements for assistance, but the improvements may be functions of different mechanisms. As another example, of 3 patients being taught to transfer from a wheelchair to a regular chair, the first may require assistance in transferring because he is so impulsive that he is unsafe, the second may require assistance because he catches his brace on the pedal of his wheelchair, while the third may require help because he forgets to lock his wheelchair. Identifying all 3 patients only in terms of amount of assistance needed may block further examination of what the patient actually does when he transfers, so that we stop thinking about the mechanisms which underlie the disturbance and the ways of eliciting the correct performance. It is of interest to note that while the concept of need for assistance has received wide acceptance as a measure of the patient's competence, the nature and conditions of need for assistance itself have not been well explicated. Amount of assistance required can be described as (1) a physical therapist's judgment of the degree of physical danger the patient risks in performing an act or (2) as the degree of support required to actually complete the act. While these two concepts overlap, they are not identical.

Despite these strictures, scaling degree of independence in terms of the amount of assistance required may be a useful, practical approach which can generate data which are clinically and statistically meaningful (Schoening and Iverson, 1968).

STATISTICAL METHODOLOGY

While the aim of this discussion is not to evaluate or examine the statistical properties of ADL scales, nevertheless certain comments on statistical methodology are worthy of mention. First, there is increasing evidence of concern with reliability of measurement (Peszczynski and Bruell, 1960). Second, there is a paucity of substantive data on validity. Gordon and Kohn (1966), in presenting their scales for ADL, argued in favor of accepting them on the grounds that the degrees of impairment which serve as reference points are related to ultimate disposition. However, data substantiating this assertion were not presented. Kelman and Muller (1962) noted that nursing home residents performed better in a rehabilitation setting than in a nursing home setting. Schoening and Iverson (1968) attempted to educe evidence for considering impairment in ADL in terms of the amount of staff time required to assist the patient. Scull *et al.* (1962) attempted to relate physician's examination of patients with patients' own statements to establish the degree of independence in a home setting following rehabilitation. The numerical properties of the scoring systems have ranged from the highly primitive to the highly sophisticated. In addition to the usual requirements for proper tests of statistical significance, the following problems are present: (1) Most authors assume that steps in ADL scales are of equal interval so that a score of 2 is twice that of 1. This assumption is not justified (Peszczynski and Bruell, 1960; Gordon and Kohn, 1966). (2) The measurement of gain in terms of raw scores and percentages is beset with many difficulties so that different ways of tabulating ADL improvement, as Kelman and Willner (1962) have demonstrated, lead to different results. (3) Few authors take into account the fact that there is a natural ceiling on the scales so that individuals who enter at a lower point on a scale have a chance for gaining more points. Some ways of coping with this problem are by equating for level of entry (Bourestom and Howard, 1968) or by dividing actual gain by maximum possible gain (Benton, Brown, and Rengler, 1951).

PROCESSES OF ACQUIRING SKILL IN ADL

Schoening (1965, 1968) and his colleagues developed a scale in which they were able to show how (1) severity of disability is related to the amount of staff time required to assist the patient; (2) the degree of improvement is related to the duration of treatment; (3) if amount of assistance offered to a patient in transfer tasks is plotted on a weekly basis, the curves for left hemiplegics differ from the curves for right hemiplegics, suggesting that although initial and final achievements may be the same, different processes are taking place.

In an unpublished study in our program, it has been demonstrated that in learning transfer tasks left hemiplegics and right hemiplegics enter and leave at about the same level. However, for left hemiplegics, improvement is related to duration of stay ($r = .43$, $p = .01$, $N = 46$);

for right hemiplegics it is not (r = .14, N = 58). Whether this is unique to our center, due to a local artifact, is unclear. It has also been noted that if one observes patients in the course of learning to transfer from a wheelchair to a regular chair, one is impressed with the complex sequence of events in a seemingly simple task. The patient must learn to steer his chair into position, lock his brakes, lift his foot pedal, move forward to the edge of his seat, stand, pivot, and sit down. While it is customary to grade the patient's performance in terms of the assistance he needs (a measure of safety), it is also possible to look at deviations in style or errors. For example, some patients forget to lock their brakes, others don't move forward, others catch the foot in the pedal, etc. As one observes these errors from week to week, a number of points become apparent. It is difficult to relate subgroups or patterns of errors to any single variable. However, it does appear that perseveration of error (defined as repeating the same mistake in more than half the trials of a given day's observation) and scatter (defined as the sum of errors in a given trial) at the first session predict how much gain in need for assistance a patient will make in his training (r = .37, r = .31, p = .01, N = 58) and how much variability there will be from week to week in right hemiplegic individuals. In this regard, the importance of perseveration as a problem in learning in aphasia has been noted by others (Tikofsky and Reynolds, 1962; Allison, 1966; Allison and Hurwitz, 1967). These relations do not occur in left hemiplegic individuals.

Looking at behavior change over time yields interesting observations. If one plots the number of regressions in performance on a weekly basis, it is clear that the number of regressions (defined as a transfer requiring greater asistance compared with those of the previous week) are correlated with the level of organicity or mental status. Individuals who show signs of mental confusion, concrete thinking, etc., regress in performance more often than individuals who are mentally intact. Furthermore, it is possible to demonstrate that when the therapist is changed (e.g., a student therapist substitutes for a senior therapist), the individual with impared mental status regresses in performance while the individual who is more intact mentally does not.

These kinds of observations suggest that investigation of learning in naturalistic circumstances, a vastly neglected field of inquiry, according to Hilgard and Bower (1966), may provide information which is important clinically and theoretically (Diller and Weinberg, 1968).

PREDICTING ADL

Since this discussion is not essentially concerned with the prediction and monitoring of the disease, I will merely note that there have been a number of successful attempts to predict the outcome of ADL training in individuals with hemiplegia. Predictions can be generated by a wide variety of measures such as age; presence of previous cerebrovascular accident; time since onset of disability; indices of neurological deficit including mental confusion, sensory deficit, and incontinence; and results of psychological tests of a performance nature. The predictions relate to success in ambulation, duration of rehabilitation treatment, and final disposition. With regard to the criteria, few studies attempt to relate different predictors to different kinds of outcomes. Yet, it is of interest to note that the retrospective study of Lee *et al.* (1958) includes a clinical rating of motivation to predict disposition. In addition, some studies demonstrate improvement in certain skill areas, e.g., transfer activities (Schoening and Iverson, 1968), while other studies show little improvement in a skill area as a result of rehabilitation, e.g., Williams' (1967) study of dressing in hemiplegia, which suggests that most patients who are competent in dressing on entering a program are competent on leaving, and those who are not competent on entering are not competent on leaving.

CHANGING BEHAVIOR IN THE CLINICAL SITUATION

Although this review is not concerned with neurophysiological or neuromuscular aspects of treatment of sensory and motor disturbances in hemiplegia, a few comments to guide the reader may be in order. Therapeutic exercises for the hemiplegic patient were known during the nineteenth century. An early regimen in this country was presented by Clayton (1924). The predominant approach until the 1960's was somewhat arbitrary with respect to the application of neurophysiological principles. Some exercises suggested a sensory facilitation rationale, but this concept was not elaborated upon. Some regimens followed the principles of normal motor development, i.e., proximal-to-distal functional return of the extremities: Exercise was emphasized at proximal joints where return was first expected. Westcott (1967) has offered a brief noncritical evaluation of this approach.

In the past decade, there has been an attempt to introduce therapeutic regimens based on neurophysiological theory. Fay (1955), Brunnstrom (1956), Bobath (1959), Kabat (1961), and Rood (1962) have certain common points: (1) in methods for facilitation and inhibition of motor activity, it is acknowledged that sensation and motion are intimately related in normal functioning, and each method uses sensory input to some degree to facilitate or inhibit movement (e.g., Rood and Kabat use cold); (2) each method is based on a postulated sequence of normal motor development; (3) each method recognizes that early motor behavior is influenced by reflex activity, and in treatment these reflex mechanisms are used to inhibit or facilitate voluntary effort; (4) each method employs important concepts of motor learning such as repetition of activity, frequency of stimulation, and use of sensory cues to facilitate learning; (5) each method focuses on the interaction of the body and its segments as a whole; (6) each method depends on the interaction between patient and therapist (Flanagan, 1967). As yet, these techniques have not been subjected to systematic comparisons. On a more elementary level, there are few data on such basic parameters of treatment as frequency, duration, carry-over of effects, and ways in which various approaches differ. Some of the common points touch on traditional and current issues in neuropsychology which we will point out later.

A number of behavioral approaches derived from styles of therapy currently prevalent in psychology have been utilized to supplement approaches based on neurophysiological considerations. These include hypnosis, task-oriented psychotherapy, and operant conditioning. Using hypnosis, Alexander (1966) has reported success in the treatment of an individual with left hemiplegia due to head trauma. In this particular case, hypnosis with techniques of relaxation was able to improve a strong component of depressive-hysterical overlay after 22 months of fixed, static disability; despite some minor residual hemiparesis and hemihypesthesia, the patient was able to return to work. Rosen and his associates were not able to find any improvement in performance in a group of hemiplegics under hypnosis who were tested on two-point touch, motor impersistence, and the Purdue Peg Board (Rosen, personal communication). However, they observed an objective gain in scores on the part of some patients and a subjective increase in sensation in other patients, so that results must be considered as inconclusive. It is of interest to note that hypnosis has been utilized successfully in an opposite way. London and Bryan (1960) were able to induce impairment of the abstract attitude by suggesting to subjects that they were brain-injured. Fromm and her coworkers (1964) were able to elicit "organic" responses to psychological tests by suggesting to the patients that they were hemiplegic and brain-damaged. It may be that hypnosis affects emotional states which influence sensory or motor functioning.

In a series of papers describing a psychotherapeutic approach to psychological problems associated with motor disturbances in disabled people, Zane (1967) suggested that individuals who fail to complete a motor act as a result of anxiety or of a symbolic misrepresentation of the demands of the act may be helped by task-oriented psychotherapy. In this procedure, the patient may perform the feared act (in the presence of the physical therapist or in his absence) with the psychotherapist at his side, eliciting his feelings and responses to the act as they unfold. With the therapist at his side, the patient feels less anxious. He is also guided to pay attention to the demands of the task rather than to some private symbolic idea. While the strong relations between neurophysiological functions and improvement in ADL performance suggest that attidudinal factors are not the critical ones, the role of close personal contact has been emphasized by every school of therapy, as indicated above. Furthermore, there are undoubtedly some patients with emotional problems who do distort what is asked of them. Finally, the deleterious effects of anxiety on a psychomotor performance in brain-injured people must be considered.

Behavior therapy, which has made a profound impact in various areas of psychology concerned with behavioral change, has been utilized to influence motor behavior of non-brain-damaged people, including feeding behavior (Allyon, 1963), pain (Fordyce, Fowler, and DeLateur, 1968), tics (Barrett, 1962), and enuresis (Wickes, 1958), as well as to influence motor behavior in a laboratory. There have been a number of attempts to improve language skills in individuals with aphasia and an attempt to improve ambulation in the case of a child with cerebral palsy (Meyerson, 1965).

The methods and purposes of behavior therapy have been well described in many texts. Even though the operant approaches are well known, let us review a typical application of the method. Generally, a number of steps are followed.

1. Defining the aberrant behavior and the response classes which are accounted with it.

2. Obtaining base rates on the emissions of aberrant behaviors while the activity is being performed. A base rate may be defined as a stable measure of activity under naturalistic conditions. Typically, the experimenter obtains behavior samples on at least three occasions to establish the reliability and limits of the response class.

3. Positively rewarding the correct response when it is emitted and ignoring all other responses. This is continued until the subject appears to have reached a plateau which may be defined as a lack of improvement in the deficit response class for 3 or more days.

4. Negatively rewarding the incorrect response until a plateau is reached.

5. Using a role-playing situation in which the examiner models the correct response while the patient watches.

6. Using token reinforcements in lieu of direct reward.

7. Having the subject reward and punish himself.

The experimenter may use other conditions which facilitate learning, e.g., stimulus enhancement, a procedure which emphasizes properties of the stimulus which distinguish it from other stimuli.

These steps are not followed in any particular sequence; each is introduced when a particular plateau is reached. To date, there are no large-scaled controlled studies which demonstrate the efficacy of these methods when applied to individuals with cerebrovascular diseases. However, Goodkin (1966) has demonstrated that it is possible to teach neurologically impaired patients to move their wheelchairs faster and to type more quickly, to teach a patient with visual spatial neglect to scan visual targets, and to teach a hemiplegic to walk better.

In evaluating the effectiveness of operant conditioning in the rehabilitation of sensory and motor disturbances in individuals with hemiplegia, one must be aware that to date, results have been presented only for individual cases, rather than for controlled studies. Operant conditioning has a number of virtues as well as some shortcomings, which should be noted. (1) It is an ingenious way of documenting occurrences in the case study method, which has, up to this point, proved unsuitable to the rigorous analysis associated with statistical and experimental methods; this may be the most valuable contribution of operant conditioning. (2) It calls attention to parameters of response classes which are generally ignored, although it leaves open the question of defining a response class which should be maintained or avoided. In this respect, it affords a great deal of flexibility, as may be seen, for example, in the forms developed by Goodkin in our program in working with physical therapists to apply operant conditioning to problems in ambulation. (3) It attempts to foster ways of emphasizing task demand variables which are apparent to the teacher, but have been neglected by the students of brain damage. (4) It attempts to translate problems into observable behaviors. The experimenter works with overt responses which can be readily seen and documented and translated into operational definitions of stimuli and responses. This last factor is largely responsible for its great popularity.

In addition to its virtues, there are a number of difficulties in applying the operant approach to a hemiplegic. (1) The hemiplegic often performs correctly under some circumstances, but not under others. He can be taught to scan his environment visually in one room, but when the room is changed, the scanning behavior ceases. To combat this difficulty in carry-over, the therapist must work not only at eliciting the correct response, but also at getting the patient to apply the correct response in other settings. The difficulty may be due to the patient's concrete thinking or to the absence of natural rather than arbitrary reinforcement (Ferster, 1967). (2) The hemiplegic patient, like other neurologically impaired people, often has many interrelated problems, including interpersonal and emotional entanglements. Selecting a sensory or motor problem for intensive effort may seem trivial to the patient who measures progress in gross terms. While denial of a loss of skill may discourage attempts to teach a patient, it can be overcome with careful interest and rapport, as Lawson's case studies and our own clinical experience (Goodkin, 1966) have shown. (3) A more serious objection arises from the fact that many students of sensorimotor behavior argue that behavioral control occurs before rather than after the act is completed. If feedback is to be effective, it must take place during either afferent or reafferent organization (Freedman, 1968).

One further instance which utilizes principles similar to those used in the previous studies might be cited. Critchley (1949) and Furmanski (1950) attempted to improve the patient's response on a task of double simultaneous stimulation (DSS) by having patients try to become aware of their errors. Furmanski reported 6 of his 12 patients overcame DSS extinction by repeated stimulation and correction of errors. However, these improvements may have been transient and specific to the occasion. Zane and Goldman (1966) attempted to teach hemiplegics to improve their performance on the face-hand test by following a systematic procedure. (1) When the patient fails, begin with the stimulus most likely to be responded to correctly by normal subjects (if face stimulation was extinguished, begin with face rather than hand; if stimulation to the unaffected hand was extinguished, begin with that hand rather than the affected one. (2) Focus on one error at a time. (3) Repeat the task with the eyes open. (4) If failure still occurs, repeat with the eyes open and suggest to the patient that he try to concentrate. (5) If he succeeds, suggest to the patient that he could probably do the task with the eyes closed. Zane and Goldman reported that they were able to improve performance in the majority of the 20 patients in their study. While it is difficult to tease out the relevant variables to which the success may be attributed, Zane and Goldman argued that the situation may well be seen as a paradigm for dealing with puzzling difficulties in walking or balancing. They attributed success to (1) hierarchic structuring of the task so that easier tasks are introduced first, (2) introducing tasks in an increasing order of difficulty, (3) offering feedback on correct performance, and (4) modifying procedures to allow for the patient's reaction to the situation.

CHANGING BEHAVIOR UNDER LABORATORY CONDITIONS

The study of behavioral change under laboratory conditions is of interest not only because of the suggestions that may be furnished for clinical practice, but also because of underlying theoretical models of neuropsychology which are at issue. We will leave the formal studies of learning in brain-damaged people to the last and review the other studies first.

Let us posit two types of approaches currently in use in neuropsychology. The first is an abilities approach which suggests that brain damage is accompanied by a selective loss in mental ability. One of the chief aims of neuropsychology is, therefore, to explicate the relations between differential losses in ability and different parameters of brain damage. Meier's paper is an excellent example of this approach which he rightly points out is an extension of a clinical neurological examination. In this approach, the underlying presumption is that of a lawfulness of behavioral deficit in terms of neuroanatomical and temporal parameters. In this approach, success and failure on varieties of tasks are used as the main indices of competence.

The second approach is oriented more toward the rehabilitation and educational aspects of deficit states. This approach is concerned with abilities and disabilities viewed in terms of strategies for their alteration. For example, it is not only concerned that a patient with left hemiplegia fails a block-design task, but also concerned with why he fails the task and under what circumstances he can be induced to succeed. The last point is at the very heart of rehabilitation, but is also related to more basic issues. In neuropsychology, the fact that successful performance may depend on the task conditions suggests that behavior is organized in a different way than is implied by a simple ability-disability concept. This is the notion behind Goldstein's use of the abstract-concrete dichotomy in which behavior present under one circumstance may not be elicited under other circumstances. Goldstein (1939) postulated that changes in the organization of behavior must reflect changes in the organization of the nervous system. It is also the notion behind Werner's postulation that patterns of disorganization of performance on the marble-board test reflect the presence of exogenous brain damage (Werner and Weir, 1956). For those who regard the work of Goldstein and Werner as somewhat dated (Reitan, 1958a; Diller and Birch, 1964), I would counter that the principle behind their arguments is valid, even if specific findings are not.

The principle has recently been restated in another context by Maier (1963), who cited the classical studies of Krechevsky on brain-injured rats. Krechevsky demonstrated that the brain-injured rats, because of their rigidity, preferred a constant path in a maze rather than a variable one. Hence, if the constant path was shorter than the variable one, the rats were superior to the non-brain-injured animals; if it was longer, they were inferior; if it was the same, they were equal. Maier suggested, therefore, that ability and performance are not the same, for performance depends on specific conditions. He then cited some of the more general conditions which might mediate the difference. These include phenomena of motivation, set, perceptual organization of the task, etc. In Maier's terms the brain-damaged person may differ from normal on the basis of different kinds of specific sensorimotor or verbal deficits, but he may also suffer from an inability to select and integrate response patterns which are within his repertoire. Brain damage, in short, not only causes deficits or disabilities, but also causes interferences with the organization of behavior.

Let us, therefore, divide laboratory studies of behavioral change in hemiplegia into two groups: those based on abilities models and those based on organization models.

STUDIES BASED ON ABILITY-DISABILITY MODELS

Fordyce and Jones (1966) have shown that the type of instruction used in solving a pegboard problem has a differential effect depending on the side of disability. Persons with right hemiplegia, for example, who characteristically perform less well on verbal than on psychomotor tasks, respond better to nonverbal than to verbal instructions, while those with left hemiplegia show an opposite effect on the Purdue Peg Board. Patients with left hemiplegia perform better under verbal than under nonverbal conditions. This would seem to have important implications for teaching.

First, it raises the question, what is the relation between competence in task performance and ability to profit from cues? Fordyce and Jones implied a clear relation. People may fail to use cues in their area of incompetence, although they use cues which tap their more intact skills. Work in progress in our own setting (Ben-Yishay *et al.*, 1970) suggests that the ability to profit from cues on a block-design task is highly related to original competence on the task. For example, if one left hemiplegic patient passed one block-design task, and a second passed five block-design tasks, then the latter would require fewer cues to solve a problem which was beyond the ability level of both of them. This finding is in accord with studies on learning of block designs in non-brain-damaged people (Budoff and Friedmann, 1964; Schubert, 1967). It is also in accord with the way acquisition of skills in ADL takes place in rehabilitation programs, i.e., by slow, progressive, stepwise increments rather than spectacular leaps. Why this should be the case is not known. The most simple explanation may be that ability to pay attention to cues depends on perceptual organization.

A second conclusion to be drawn from Fordyce and Jones' study is that in training it is better to utilize a channel which is more intact than one which is more impaired. This finding documents a clinical impression of Belmont's (1957), as well as our own clinical impressions. However, there are no data on how much variance a given channel of communication actually contributes in a live clinical setting. For example, many therapists offer little formal instruction in teaching on ADL skill since the task demands are obvious. The instruction usually comes in the correction of errors.

While the principle of utilizing the intact channel may be useful, the demands of the task must also be analyzed in terms of the abilities required to complete it. For example, several years ago it was shown that right and left hemiplegics did about equally well in solving the well-known oddity problem, such as the kind used by Harlow to study learning sets. The same finding held true when the rewards were reversed so that one of the even stimuli was now correct and the odd stimulus was incorrect. In short, in a reversal learning situation, right hemiplegics and left hemiplegics perform about equally well. In noting the difference between the original learning and the reversal learning, it was discovered that improvement in the reversal situation held different contingencies for right and left hemiplegics. For left hemiplegics improvement was related to the rod test, a spatial perceptual task which yielded impaired performance in left hemiplegic patients, while improvement in the reversal situation was related to a verbal test in right hemiplegic patients, most of whom were aphasic. From this one can conclude that (1) two patients can pass or fail the same task for different reasons, so that while it is possible that a right hemiplegic and a left hemiplegic learn to transfer equally well, it is also possible that they do this for different reasons, and (2) improvement is not dependent on the intact modality as much as on the impaired modality. This last is an important principle since rehabilitation has been thought of in terms of utilizing the patient's assets. The study suggests that, in the case of hemiplegics, in certain tasks defects cannot be ignored (Diller and Weinberg, 1968).

One final point suggested by the Fordyce and Jones study concerns time as a parameter of competence. Costa and Vaughn (1962) have suggested that when time limits are increased for a block-design task, normal individuals and right hemiplegics improve their performance, while left hemiplegics do not. Similarly, Diller and Weinberg (1968) noted that in performing visual cancellation tasks, left hemiplegics are much quicker than right hemiplegics. It follows from this that increasing time limits would help the right hemiplegic, who tends to be slow, but would not improve the performance of the left hemiplegic, who works too quickly. An interesting clinical observation here is that if one tells the left hemiplegic patient to slow down, he improves his performance. This is not the case for the right hemiplegic. In the latter instance, one might suspect that the patient is slowed down by his difficulty in verbal self-rehearsal which may be associated with aphasia.

STUDIES BASED ON ORGANIZATION MODELS

There is an interesting series of studies designed to investigate the theory that behavioral organization of brain-damaged individuals differs from that of non-brain-damaged individuals. The method for demonstrating this has been to vary the task conditions and demonstrate that under the changed circumstances the brain-damaged individual improves until he equals or exceeds the normal person, whereas the normal person does not improve or deteriorates. A review of some of these phenomena is of both theoretical and clinical interest.

Perhaps the prime examples of this approach in the field of hemiplegia are three series of studies launched by Birch and his associates. In each of these studies, Birch was not interested in the therapeutic effect of the experiment. His major point was that disorganization of behavior is lawful and illuminates the way in which the central nervous system operates.

In the first series, Birch *et al.* (1961) argue that if brain damage leads to a regression in behavior, one can expect behavior dependent on intersensory organization to be impaired more rapidly than behavior based on intrasensory organization, in accordance with Sherrington's views of the development of the nervous system. It follows, therefore, that if one introduces an intrasensory task, one might improve the behavior of the hemiplegic, but not that of a normal person. This indeed appeared to occur. When a luminous frame was introduced after the patient's response to the luminous rod, this apparently had a salutary effect on hemiplegic patients, but not on controls. Presumably, judgment of a luminous rod is dependent on both visual and postural cues, an intersensory task. The frame helps to define the task as intrasensory. A therapist would, therefore, attempt to present tasks within the same sensory modality if he wanted to improve a patient's behavior.

In another series of studies based on similar reasoning (Bortner and Birch, 1960), it has been demonstrated that left hemiplegics who fail on a block-design test can complete the task when it is presented as a multiple-choice test. Presumably this is because visual discrimination precedes visual execution in the course of normal development so that it is more refractory to impairment due to central nervous system damage. An alternative interpretation and a brief review of studies in this area have recently been presented (Domrath, 1968). In accordance with the reasoning of Birch and Bortner, a patient who fails a constructional task might well be presented with a series of visual discrimination tasks before proceeding further.

In another series of studies (Belmont, Birch, and Karp, 1966; Birch, Belmont, and Karp, 1967) it has been suggested that the so-called phenomenon of extinction in double simultaneous stimulation occurs because (1) there is a lag in the speed of transmission of the stimuli on the impaired side, and (2) there is a slowness of recovery from the presentation of preceding stimuli on the impaired side. If this reasoning is correct, one can show that in instances when the stimulus on the impaired side is made more intense or longer, or precedes the stimulus on the intact side, the stimulus on the impaired side is recognized and even extinguishes stimuli on the intact side. The sensory delay theory suggests that under certain circumstances, presenting a stimulus on the impaired side may elicit a better response in a therapeutic situation than presenting it on the intact side. This is in contrast to the widely held opinion that patients should generally receive instruction and stimulation from their intact side.

A finding pertinent to a consideration of the effects of asymmetric stimulation is that bilateral movement in hemiplegia deteriorates the performance of both healthy and impaired hands. Hausmanowa-Petrusewicz (1959) found this to be the case in a bulb-squeezing task sensitive to strength of movement. The effect appears when the movement is passive as well as when it is active. This finding confirms an earlier study of Cohn (1951), who found that simultaneous bilateral pronation and supernation impaired the performance of the good hand and did not improve the affected one. The studies suggest that in rehabilitation activities, movements are not necessarily more effective under bilateral conditions. In a series of 5 cases, we were able to observe that a hemiplegic individual performed well when the therapist provided assistance by holding a piece of cloth on the table while the patient buttoned with his unaffected hand. However, when the patient used his impaired hand as a weight or stabilizer, performance deteriorated.

There are other instances wherein the nature of the task condition influences performance with regard to rehabilitation procedures. Lawson (1962) reported teaching reading to 2 individuals with left hemiplegia by presenting materials from a right to left direction, rather than the traditional left to right. Similarly, we have noted that left hemiplegic individuals show aberrant scanning patterns, with preferences from right to left instead of left to right. We were unable to note aberrant styles in right hemiplegics. In this connection it should be noted that there is a growing literature on scanning habits in normal individuals, with some suggestion that normal individuals are more efficient in recognizing materials presented in the right side of space than those presented in the left side of space (Heron, 1957; Wyke and Ettlinger, 1961; Harcum, 1967). The nature of the task also may influence side of presentation. For example, in teaching a hemiplegic to transfer from a wheelchair to a regular chair, one notices that different trainers utilize different approaches. In some programs, the patient is taught to line up the wheelchair so that the regular chair is on the impaired side, and the patient pivots from his unaffected side to his affected side. In other programs, the opposite is taught so that the patient leads with his unimpaired side.

Problems associated with visual field defect and neglect can also be examined from the standpoint of manipulation of task conditions. These problems have received a great deal of attention from psychologists and neurologists (Denny-Brown, 1958) during the past 2 decades, but there have been few controlled or clinical studies attempting to remedy these problems in rehabilitation settings. In this regard two series of studies appear pertinent. The first is a project undertaken by Poppelreuter (1917) which demonstrates that for some patients with hemianopia visual forms are "completed" across blind sections of the visual field. When a figure is exposed on the tachistoscope screen so that it overlaps a blind part of the visual field, the patients still report seeing the whole figure, though this is objectively impossible. Since not all patients with hemianopia react this way, there have been a number of attempts to discover why. Some have suggested that completion occurs in patients with residual vision; others that it occurs in mentally confused patients. Warrington (1962) suggested that it is associated primarily with parietal lobe damage and unawareness of field defect. The study is of interest because of the paucity of attempts to investigate the consequences of visual field defects for rehabilitation and establish a taxonomy of responses to defects from the standpoint of training procedures. The second series of studies is pertinent not only because of its concern with spatial inattention, but also because it demonstrates again that a patient with brain damage can improve his performance in situations where a non-brain-damaged person does not. This series of studies (Williams *et al.*, 1956; Yates, 1956; Hovey, 1961; Williams, Gieseking, and Lubin, 1961) initiated by Shapiro (1953), has demonstrated that although a brain-damaged patient shows more rotations than does a normal patient in block-design tasks, this inferiority can be remedied if the patient performs the block design while viewing the target through a pinhole of light. The theory has been proposed that peripheral intrasensory stimulation serves as a distraction in the brain-damaged individual, while in the normal person peripheral stimuli serve to facilitate performance. This line of reasoning is in accord with the notion of attempting to reduce all stimulation except the most essential in teaching a brain-damaged person to master a task. Gilliatt and Pratt (1952) presented one of several reports which indicate that patients can sometimes perform better with their eyes closed than with their eyes open.

THE STUDY OF LEARNING IN INDIVIDUALS WITH BRAIN DAMAGE

While most of the laboratory interest in brain-damaged patients has been in the area of perception, a number of studies examine dimensions of learning which bear on behavior change in brain-damaged people. These include studies of stimulus generalization, massed versus spaced practice, attention, types of instruction, and discrimination learning.

Stimulus generalization refers to the situation where a response previously trained to be elicited by a given stimulus, can also be elicited by stimuli similar to the original. It is said to occupy a central place in phenomena of learning (Mednick and Freedman, 1960). Mednick (1955) and Carson (1958) have presented evidence that brain-damaged people (including hemiplegics) in contrast to schizophrenics and normal individuals, undergeneralize. This holds for spatial tasks (Mednick, 1955) as well as verbal tasks (Carson, 1958). The phenomenon may be postulated to account for the concrete behavior of brain-damaged people in terms of learning theory. It would explain, for instance, why a patient who learns under one set of circumstances fails under another set of circumstances. It is also possible that under certain circumstances where stimuli compete with each other, the inability to generalize may be a virtue, for example, in a sheltered workshop, where the ability to carry out repetitive activities is an asset.

While the role of practice in learning psychomotor skills has been of central concern to students of motor skills and of learning, there are few studies of the effects of practice in brain-damaged people. Franz (1915), an early student of the problem, felt that hemiplegics can learn motor skills and on this basis argued for early reeducation of hemiplegics. Van Buskirk (1954) administered a battery of simple motor tasks to a series of 39 hemiplegics. The tests were repeated daily, and the weekly averages were used to study performance curves. The tests consisted of tapping, alternate pronation and supernation of the forearm, and speed of elbow flexion. It was determined that although dexterity was decreased on the paretic side, the ability to learn remained equal to that of the nonparetic side. "Learning" on both paretic and nonparetic sides appeared more satisfactory during the first 2 months after the onset of the disability. With increasing time, the rate of learning declined. Results are attributed to restitution of function following brain injury—a spontaneous process.

Huse and Parsons (1965), who utilized a pursuit motor task as a way of studying the acquisition of habits in the brain-damaged, found that brain-damaged individuals were inferior in level of performance and rate of improvement to a control group under massed and spaced practice conditions, but no differential deficit due to conditions was present. The more severe the brain damage, the greater the lag in both performance and rate of improvement. There appears to be no differences between patients with right and with left hemispheric lesions. Level of sensorimotor dysfunction appears to be the critical variable.

Problems in attention have recently assumed importance in investigative and clinical work. On the theoretical side, this interest has been fostered by several converging streams of influence from experimenters who have been looking at different phenomena. First, the English psychologists have been concerned with phenomena of vigilance associated with the monitoring of signals over a period of time. This line of query has led to viewing attention from an information-processing standpoint (Broadbent, 1957; Welford and Birren, 1965). Second, neurophysiologists have been concerned with phenomena of arousal, sleeping, and activation (Hernandez-Peon, 1964). Third, students of cognitive development have shown concern with attentional phenomena. For example, Gestalt psychology classically translated the problem of selection-inhibition into a problem of figure-ground (Teuber, 1959). Students of Piaget, concerned with the development of enduring cognitive structures, have spoken of mental development in terms of the ability to take in more than one stimulus at a time or the ability to take in one stimulus while keeping in mind another one—decentering (Feffer, 1967). Other theorists have distinguished between broad and narrow attention (Wachtel, 1967) and between attention span (the number of stimulus elements) and scan (the ability to actively search out information in the environment). Whether the different phenomena associated with attention are the same or different is far from academic when considered in terms of hemiplegia.

For example, does a patient who has difficulty in a psychomotor task fail to notice the cue? Does he notice the cue but lose track of it, as he has to respond to a series of cues or to several simultaneous cues? Does he fail to maintain an active search for cues to help monitor his performance (Rosvold *et al.*, 1956; Gibson, 1962)? These questions were suggested to us when we first noticed that some patients did not seem to be looking at the therapist during the course of instruction. Others appeared to be responding to irrelevant cues.

With regard to individuals with brain damage, Hunt and Cofer (1944) reviewed some of the early work in the field in which reaction-time measures have been utilized to indicate a lag in response in brain-damaged individuals. Benton and his associates have utilized this classical tool in a series of studies yielding the following findings: (1) Brain-damaged people are impaired in both simple and choice reaction time (Blackburn and Benton, 1955). (2) There are no great differences between normal and brain-damaged people with regard to the effects of practice (Benton and Blackburn, 1957). (3) Patients with right hemispheric involvement are significantly quicker in responding with the right hand than in responding with the left hand, but there are no clear-cut asymmetric differences in patients with left hemispheric involvement (Benton and Joynt, 1959). (4) The use of motivating instructions is moderately helpful. "Standard," "relaxing," and "urging" instructions (Blackburn, 1958) and "success" and "failure" instructions (Shankweiler, 1959) affect performance but only to a minor degree.

Benton *et al.* (1962) found that in a serial reaction-time task, both brain-damaged and schizophrenic patients had longer reaction times to stimuli preceded by a different stimulus than to stimuli preceded by the same stimulus. In the case of the brain-damaged group, the degree of retardation in reaction time to visual stimuli preceded by an auditory stimulus, was significantly greater than in controls. Patients with diffuse or bilateral cerebral disease showed a significantly larger cross-modal integration retardation than control patients; patients with focal lesions did not. While schizophrenics showed a cross-modal retardation, this occurred when the visual stimulus preceded the auditory stimulus. These results are in contrast with those of Lawson, McGhie, and Chapman (1967), who found schizophrenic patients, temporal lobe epileptics, and arteriosclerotic patients more distractible in a short-term auditory memory test than normal and paranoid individuals. An analogous reaction was not found in a test of visual distractibility. It should also be noted that visual retention of digits under nondistracting conditions was more impaired than auditory retention in schizophrenic and arteriosclerotic patients.

In our own program we have found that responses to attentional tasks yield interesting findings with regard to right and left hemiplegia. For example, there appear to be modality differences in scanning tasks but not in span tasks. Right hemiplegics do quite poorly in an auditory cancellation task where they are required to raise their hand to a designated digit or letter. Conversely, they do relatively well when they are required to cross out the same designated letter or digit presented visually as a visual cancellation task. On tasks of auditory digit span and visual digit span, left hemiplegics are superior to the right hemiplegics. The most reasonable assumption is that span tests require some kind of self-rehearsal and that this ability is impaired in individuals with right hemiplegia. It is of further interest to note that when patients are asked to translate a sound pattern (e.g., taps) into a visual pattern (e.g., dots displayed on a card) both groups perform equally well. However, performance in the right hemiplegic group is highly correlated with auditory cancellation and digit span (verbal and visual), while performance in the left hemiplegic group is correlated with visual cancellation. An impaired modality operates in insidious ways.

A more precise statement of the nature of the attentional difficulty may guide us in relating specific kinds of impairments in attention to specific neuroanatomic parameters. In this regard, McDonald and Burns (1964) have suggested performance deficit on a vigilance task is associated with lesions of the basal ganglia. Such improved understanding also may yield insight into retraining procedures. For example, it might be argued that the gains in performance of a skill are associated with gains in attention and that certain parameters of attention are the underlying structural variables being treated in a retraining situation. We have found that gains on a functional communication profile in aphasia are related to gains in attention span as measured by a digit span test. Analogous reasoning may be applied to the gains in sensorimotor skills. Another way of stating this is that the patient's deficit is primarily in one or more parameters of attention and that what we treat are these parameters.

What is the effect of training in visual versus tactile sense modality? According to Battersby, Krieger, and Bender (1955), learning is equally impaired in either modality and appears to be dependent on degree of general mental defect associated with organic mental syndrome. Furthermore, the locus of the brain damage appears to be irrelevant. However, it should be noted that the patients studied had cerebral tumors. Milner (1954), working with patients who had undergone cerebral excisions for removal of epileptogenic scar tissue, found somewhat different results.

In general, however, some of the major issues in learning theory or in the formal parameters of learning have received little systematic attention, from either a clinical or an experimental point of view. For example, which types of practice are more effective, whole task or part task? What is the effect of mental rehearsal? What is the effect of introducing teaching systems to help the individual monitor his own performance more accurately? What is the role of transfer? In setting up a teaching program, a physical therapist must ask himself the following questions: (1) How can the task be broken down into meaningful units? (2) How long should trials be? (3) How many trials should be offered in 1 day? (4) How many rest periods should be provided and how often? (Cross, 1967).

VOCATIONAL REHABILITATION

Estimates of return to work by hemiplegic patients following rehabilitation have ranged from 5 per cent (Knapp, 1959) to 40 per cent (Lee *et al.*, 1958). However, it is difficult to make generalizations since many of the more optimistic results pertain to patients referred to vocational, rather than medical, rehabilitation programs. These patients tend to be younger and more oriented to return to work. Among the factors which appear relevant is social class, which may affect the outcome in two major ways: (1) social class is obviously related to occupational history, occupational skills, and opportunity; (2) social class is related to critical interpersonal and familial factors, e.g., whether the individual has a home to return to following rehabilitation (Lee *et al.*, 1958). In a retrospective follow-up study, Lee (1958) found that sensory and neurologic deficits did not play a great role in successful vocational adjustment. However, Knapp (1959) argued that in left hemiplegic individuals, only 2 of 12 who were judged employable were actually working, while 6 of 11 right hemiplegics judged employable were actually working. Howard (1960) reported some success in the use of a sheltered workshop to increase employability in a series of hard core unemployed hemiplegics aged 16 to 55. Highland View Hospital in Cleveland utilized a sheltered workshop in a public hospital setting for hemiplegics. A special battery of tests, thought to be sensitive to the vocational activities of a hemiplegic, was devised (Thomas, Spangler, and Izutsu, 1961) as well as a rating scale method for evaluating adjustment. Standard vocational tests are often not applicable for this population group. Furthermore, clinical experience suggests that job sample approaches have proved much more effective than vocational tests. The Purdue Peg Board, a well-known vocational test, has been used to assess the presence of cerebral damage in hemiplegia (Costa *et al.*, 1963).

The vocational placement of the hemiplegic patient depends not only on neurological, psychological, and familial factors, but also on the particular industry, e.g., the medical policy of the company, its size, the nature of additional demands of job-related tasks, and attitudes of personnel (Howard, 1960; Panza, 1966).

DIRECTIONS FOR FUTURE RESEARCH

In seeking guide lines for future research, it may be helpful to consider different models which may be used as frameworks. We can use these models to categorize research ideas or to guide our thinking.

THE AD HOC APPROACHES

By this is meant deliberately not formulating or imposing specific directions, but rather following up hopeful lines of investigation as they develop. Each research proposal must be judged in terms of a best fit of standards of rigor, aptness, and feasibility, and relevance to the current state of its subfield of inquiry. This approach avoids the difficulty of deciding which research proposals to investigate with the limited funds available. Indeed it would be totally within the spirit of rehabilitation to work with what is available and try to make the best of it.

THE APPLICATION OF MODELS FROM OTHER FIELDS OF INQUIRY

Three kinds of research models used in other fields might be applied to investigation of psychomotor and vocational rehabilitation: (1) a disease model, (2) a packaging-and-delivery-of-services model, and (3) a treatment model. The disease model will be considered by others at this workshop and the packaging-and-delivery-of-services model is not appropriate for this workshop. Let us, therefore, consider the treatment model.

Psychotherapy research has many points in common with rehabilitation research. Among the questions common to both fields are whether therapy works, how to measure outcomes, what procedures are most effective, and what patients can benefit from treatment. Indeed, it has been noted that the typical middle-class, well-educated, young, white American, who is the best candidate for psychotherapy, is also the best candidate for rehabilitation. On the basis of this model, research in sensorimotor rehabilitation of hemiplegics can be discussed in terms of patient variables, process variables, and outcome variables. We can ask: Who is the patient in terms of social, neurological, and psychological parameters? How can we best develop strategies for identifying what we treat and how we go about treating? How do we measure the success of these efforts from the standpoint of both the individual and the community? To follow this parallel a bit further, in psychotherapy the current fashion is to take a hard look at process, since earlier studies of outcome have proved so indecisive that advocates of psychotherapy remain unconvinced by studies showing negative results while critics are skeptical of those showing positive results.

In the field of rehabilitation there has been little articulation among the domains of who is the patient, what is the treatment, and what is the result. Furthermore, as the foregoing review has indicated, there are many gaps within each of these domains. It is my impression that perhaps the weakest area of systematic inquiry is in the domain of process: What does a rehabilitation worker do with a hemiplegic patient? Why does he do it?

ROLE OF BASIC RESEARCH

Future research in rehabilitation must include basic as well as applied research. There is an obvious need for gathering normative data, trying to understand mechanisms of dysfunction and recuperation, relating services to a clearer understanding of mechanisms, and developing rational ways of packaging services.

CONCLUSION

In reviewing the current status of behavioral aspect of sensory and motor changes in the vocational rehabilitation of hemiplegia, I have focused on the study of self-care activities as manifested in the performances included in ADL inventories. This field shows an increasing concern with the methodological aspects of defining and developing ADL scales. Among the important consequences of this development is the fact that we are on the threshold of being able to describe what happens when a patient improves in ADL performances and to predict his success in mastering ADL. It should, therefore, be possible to set up criteria not only for the success of individual patients, but also for the success of treatment programs. In reviewing approaches to changing sensory and motor behavior in clinical situations which are derived from current branches of psychology (psychotherapy, hypnosis, operant conditioning), it has been shown that work in this area is still largely on the case study, exploratory level. Operant conditioning, however, promises to be useful both in clinical work and in improving styles of teaching. The laboratory studies of behavioral change may be useful in permitting analysis of patient disability and clarifying mechanisms of central nervous system disturbance which might be used in facilitating changes in behavior. However, these studies have not as yet had any serious impact on the management of patients in a clinical way. Some considerations of the implications of different laboratory approaches and a brief picture of the current status of vocational rehabilitation have been presented.

PRESENTATION 12

Glenn Gullickson, Jr.

In the management of the disabled person, the goal is that he will learn to perform at the maximum level of his remaining capabilities. This level may vary all the way from almost complete dependence to vocational independence. For a majority of hemiplegic patients the level of independent function they can achieve lies between these two extremes, and the usual rehabilitation goal is independence in the essential activities of daily living (ADL).

Diller has presented a thorough summary of the development, problems, and uses of ADL scales and ADL training in rehabilitation. The functional evaluation concept typified by the ADL scales developed because of a need for an objective system of evaluating motor functioning. The multiplicity of functional rating scales in use today, ranging from simple quantifications of the amount of care needed to detailed and cumbersome descriptions of the patient's ability in every activity in which he engages, indicates that more development is necessary in the concept of functional evaluation and measurement.

ADL tests are designed to assess a patient's physical capacity to care for himself. Also, as Schoening and Iverson (1968) note, measures are needed of the patient's emotional capacity to function within his environment, or the manner in which he interacts on a social level within his environment. One attempt to develop such a behavior rating scale for hemiplegics is that initiated by Bourestom and being continued by Iverson at the Kenny Rehabilitation Institute. Their criteria (Bourestom, 1967) for an adequate behavior rating scale are:

1. The scale should cover only those aspects of behavior which rehabilitation therapists purport to influence, which they have opportunity to observe, and which they consider when evaluating improvement of a hemiplegic patient.
2. The scale should cover only those aspects of behavior that can be objectively rated in a short period of time by raters with minimal training in the use of the scale.

3. The scale should yield a quantifiable measure of behavior.

Because some aspects of behavior are more relevant to the observations of a particular discipline, three scales have been developed with 59 items for nursing, 56 items for occupational therapy, and 49 items for physical therapy, with 29 items the same on all three forms. An example of the content is that in the nursing form, where 13 areas of behavior are considered: cooperation, appearance, awareness, initiative, emotional reaction, socialization, memory, orientation, alertness, pain, judgment, dependency, and hostility. For each of the areas, varying numbers of items have been developed to describe or define the behavior observed. For example, under "awareness," patients are rated as:

1. Able to locate wheelchair brakes on impaired side
2. Aware of foot pedal on wheelchair on impaired side
3. Aware of impaired arm
4. Aware of impaired leg
5. Aware of objects or obstacles on affected side

Under "socialization," patients are rated as:

1. Extends greeting to others verbally and/or through gestures
2. Seeks out the company of others
3. Avoids the company of others
4. Responds to nurse's interest in family, friends, occupation, avocations, or other social matters
5. Eager to see family, friends, or other visitors

Each item is rated on a 4-point scale as follows: definitely characteristic, usually characteristic, not usually characteristic, and definitely not characteristic; where there is insufficient information, the rating is not applicable or cannot say. In investigating the reliability of the behavior adjustment rating scale, the authors found that the correlations for both admission and discharge ratings ranged from .60 to .79, with the data indicating little variation in rater agreement, whether within the three disciplines or between them. They concluded that the behavior of elderly brain-damaged patients can be defined and recorded numerically with objectivity, reliability, and simplicity.

As Diller notes there have been a number of studies on predicting the outcome of rehabilitation of the hemiplegic patient. With the increasing cost of rehabilitation, it is increasingly important that there be developed well-defined outcome criteria and objective predictors of the results to be expected from a rehabilitation regimen for a particular patient. A major and ongoing attempt at establishing criteria for assessing the probable benefits of rehabilitation for hemiplegic patients is a research project of the Kenny Rehabilitation Institute entitled "Rehabilitative Predictors in Cerebrovascular Disease." This study has attempted to elicit, from the information available at the time of a stroke patient's admission, those items of information most prognostic of rehabilitation outcome. The objective criteria for outcome used in the study are the Kenny Self-Care Score for physical abilities, the behavioral adjustment score previously mentioned, and the Taylor Functional Communication Profile for measuring communication ability. In predicting a patient's self-care status they have found that out of 250 original variables, the following are the most important:

1. Duration since onset
2. Level of consciousness during acute phase
3. Diastolic blood pressure
4. Degree of bladder continence versus incontinence
5. Self-care score at admission
6. Neurological involvement, right- or left-sided
   a. Left hemiparesis
      Absence of pain and temperature sensation
      Hyperactive deep tendon reflexes, right triceps and patella
      Limitation of abductors, right shoulder
   b. Right hemiparesis
      Right field deficit
      Diminished gag reflexes
7. Severity of visumotor disturbances
8. Impairment of voice quality
9. Scale score on the Minnesota Multiphasic Personality Inventory
10. Score on the Picture Arrangement Subtest of the Wechsler Adult Intelligence Scale

From studies such as this one it will be possible to identify measurable patient characteristics related to rehabilitation outcome. With some quantification of the extent of these relations, it may become possible to manipulate certain of the factors influencing outcome and achieve the maximum optimal outcome in stroke rehabilitation.

Diller has noted the introduction during the past 20 years of a number of physical therapy techniques which are grouped together as neuromuscular facilitation. For additional information about them, the reader is referred to two review articles in *Rehabilitation Literature* for April 1954 and June 1959. A few general comments should be made about these techniques for retraining the hemiplegic patient. To some extent they have assumed the character of sectarian dogma, and each has come to be looked upon as a special system of physical therapy. Particularly pertinent at this time is the applied consequence of the theory that an individual's motor functioning is organized on different developmental levels so that in retraining a patient should learn to swim and crawl before relearning to walk. Controlled studies have not been done, and there is a real question whether recovery is more rapid with these complex techniques than with the more standard physical therapy techniques such as active assistive exercise. It seems best to view these techniques as presenting working hypotheses for further research.

Behavior modification is a new therapeutic tool for rehabilitation. Diller has summarized the prospects for the use of the technique in the rehabilitation of hemiplegics as well as some of the problems of using it with these patients. From a practical standpoint it should also be noted that another problem in using operant conditioning techniques with a specific patient is that it requires the participation of almost all the staff who have contact with that patient. Obtaining and maintaining the cooperation, if not enthusiastic participation, of all staff members in a center can be difficult though certainly not impossible.

The application of behavior modification approaches in a rehabilitation setting could be expected to improve the efficiency and effectiveness of the rehabilitation process. However, controlled research comparing existing procedures and techniques with those instituted under behavior modification will be needed.

As previously noted, the usual rehabilitation goal for most stroke patients is achieving independence in the activities of daily living, whereas the goal for most other rehabilitation center patients is vocational placement. In spite of the extensive programs which can be provided for the hemiplegic, vocational rehabilitation continues to be most difficult. In the state-federal vocational rehabilitation program about 1,000 stroke patients are rehabilitated yearly from an estimated 250,000 in the age group 25 to 64 years.

There are a number of reasons for these poor results within the employable age group. Residual motor function, but even more important residual intellectual function, are determinants of employability. The behavioral differences between right and left hemiplegics have been described. The practicality of these differences are that the vocational potential of right hemiplegics with aphasia may be underestimated, whereas the vocational potential of left hemiplegic with perceptual deficits is overestimated. Placement statistics for right and left hemiplegics are limited. Diller quotes Knapp's findings of the low figure for employed left hemiplegics.

In addition to the physical and behavioral deficits of the hemiplegic patient are major social dislocations for the patient and his family. Of importance for the eventual employment of the potentially employable hemiplegic is his return to his family and familiar environment.

In the evaluation of the employment potential and production capacities of the hemiplegic, it has been found that the best indications are obtained from actual work evaluations with necessary training provided. Interestingly, in the case of the hemiplegic housewife, it was found by Johannsen that homemaking training, which is usually provided in most center programs, added little to a patient's rehabilitation except a slight effect on proficiency.

PRESENTATION 13

Peter H. Stern
Fletcher H. McDowell

There is a trend in medicine to develop clinical examination procedures which will add quantitative data to the usual qualitative observations. We believe that clinicians involved in rehabilitation medicine would welcome a method which allows objective and unbiased evaluation of patients' responses to the variety of rehabilitative techniques used. We have developed a test battery to provide objective measurements of neuromuscular dysfunction in patients with stroke. This battery includes the tests concerned with sensation and vision as used by Tourtellotte *et al.* (1965) in their study evaluating the response of patients with multiple sclerosis to ACTH.

In order to establish correlations between our method of quantitative testing and function, the Numerical Self-Care Scoring System of the Kenny Institute of Rehabilitation was used. For aphasic patients we adopted the Taylor Functional Communication Profile. In spite of their established validity and reliability, both these latter tests are still qualitative, subjective procedures. Nevertheless, we found it important to add them to the quantitative battery in order to establish a more comprehensive profile of the patient with stroke. The tests used in our study were as follows:

1. Motility tests
   a. Tapping rate for 60 seconds, distal muscles of hands and feet
   b. Tapping rate and accuracy for 30 seconds, proximal muscles of arms and legs

   A specially designed motility recorder was used for scoring the motility index
2. Strength
   a. Knee extensors
   b. Knee flexors

   The Cybex torque dynamometer was used for this test.

3. Sensory perception
   a. Vibrometry (finger and toe)
   b. Two-point discrimination (index finger only)
4. Vision
   a. Visual acuity
   b. Visual fields
5. Functional evaluations
   a. KIR Numerical Self-Care Scoring System
   b. Taylor Functional Communication Profile

DESCRIPTION OF THE TEST BATTERY

MOTILITY

The motility recorder, and the motility index as its scoring system, were developed to allow quantitative observations of motility change in patients with stroke over time and under the influence of rehabilitation procedures. Utilizing this system, the hemiplegic side can be compared with the nonhemiplegic side, and each side can also be compared with a normal population group. Normative values have been established in previous standardization studies.

Description of Apparatus and Methodology. The motility recorder, the details of methodology, and the standardization have been previously described (Stern *et al.*, 1969). The procedure involves two tests each for the upper and lower extremities of the affected and unaffected sides. The patient is requested to activate, by tapping, targets which trip electrical counters controlled by program timers. The patient's ability to perform rapid, repetitive motions can be scored numerically over time. The apparatus tests the performance of distal muscle groups in the hands and feet and the performance of the proximal muscle groups of shoulders and arms, thighs, and hips. Since the only intelligence required is the ability to follow simple commands, it is possible to test patients even in the presence of some degree of aphasia or dementia. Eight subtests are necessary to complete the total test.

Measurement of Motility Defects. In order to score more easily the patient's performance on the motility recorder, a motility index was developed to reduce the number of scores from 8 to 1. The motility index is defined as the function of the 8 subscores mentioned and has the property that a normal motility score is 0 and less than normal motility has a negative score. The motility index associated with total hemiplegia is about —22. Bilateral involvement is indicated by an index below —22, and total quadriplegia scores about —44. In order to compile tests results, the following formula was developed:

$$MI = 1/10\, X_1 + X_2 + X_3 + X_4 + 2X_5 + X_6 + X_7 + X_8 - 448$$

X_1 through X_4 represents the scores for the tests involving distal muscles of hands and feet. X_5 through X_8 represents scores for the tests involving proximal muscles of shoulders and arms, thighs, and hips. The number 448 is the constant obtained from the average scores of a population of 150 normal subjects used in standardizing the test. Subindices can be computed for each side of the body separately; the respective standardizing constants for the right and left sides of the body are 223 and 215. The motility index for total performance, as well as the subindices, are determined upon admission, at weekly intervals, and at discharge.

STRENGTH

The determination of muscle strength, particularly in patients with upper motor neuron involvement, is difficult. The methods determining muscle strength currently in use are either not quantitative or not suitable for clinical use (cf. Beasley, 1956; Daniels, Williams, and Worthingham, 1956). As standardization procedures are practically impossible, owing to the great variability among subjects, in our study the strength of the involved side is compared with that of the uninvolved side.

Apparatus and Methodology. The Cybex torque dynamometer is used to record the strength of both knee extensor and flexor muscle groups. This commercially available equipment measures strength applied at a set constant speed against variable resistance. Torque, in foot-pounds, is recorded as the measure of strength. The dynamometer is attached to a modified plinth with a specially designed back rest. A support under the thigh as well as provisions for strapping the patient down permits strength measurement of the functionally isolated quadriceps and hamstring muscles. Using a constant speed of 2 rpm, the strength of the knee extensors and flexors of both the involved and uninvolved sides is tested. The best of three trials is used as the score. Measurements are takn upon admission, at weekly intervals, and upon discharge.

SENSATION

Vibrometry. For this test, a Biothesiometer (Model PVD), which vibrates at 120 cps in the range from 0 to 50 μ, is used. The test is performed by placing the pad of the index finger on the vibrator with the fingerprint whorl over the center of the vibrator. In addition, the vibrator is positioned at the base of the first toe on the joint interspace. The subject is first given a recognizable stimulus. Then the amplitude of vibration is increased gradually by increasing the voltage evenly and slowly. The subject is asked to report the first perception (threshold) of vibration. The voltage level at threshold is then recorded. This procedure is repeated three times. The threshold values are converted to microns and averaged to arrive at a score. The test is performed on both the involved and uninvolved sides.

Two-Point Versus One-Point Perception. For this test, a Sweet's two-point compass calibrated in millimeters is used. The test is performed on the index finger of the involved and uninvolved sides. The subject is first given a recognizable stimulus of greater than 10 mm on the index finger pad at the center of the fingerprint whorl. The stimulus is decreased by 1 mm per trial until the subject gives three consecutive responses of perceiving one point at the same measurement.

VISION

Visual Acuity. The standard Snellen Visual Acuity Test at 20 ft is used, measuring the corrected and uncorrected vision in each eye.

Visual Fields. To determine the visual field, we employ the Harrington-Flocks Field Screener, which presents tachistoscopic visual stimuli covering the entire visual field. Responses are recorded by mapping out omissions in the presence or absence of a visual field defect. The test is done upon admission and is repeated only if changes are noted by clinical observation.

FUNCTIONAL EVALUATIONS

KIR Numerical Self-Care Scoring System. The Kenny self-care evaluation procedure is employed. Three different categories of raters are used. The test is performed upon admission, at biweekly intervals, and at discharge. The details of the procedure as published by Schoening *et al.* (1965) are strictly adhered to according to the definitions contained in the rater's manual. In this study, nurses rate all items except walking on stairs. Occupational therapists rate all items except stair-climbing and items concerned with personal hygiene, i.e., bowel and bladder programs and perineal care. Physical therapists rate only transfer and locomotion activities including stair-climbing. The scoring is recorded on the KIR Self-Care Form, which uses a 5-point scoring continuum from 0 through 4 for each of 17 self-care activities. The final self-care scores range from 0 to 24 points. Occasionally, interrater discrepancies are observed and are averaged to obtain a reasonable estimate of performance.

Taylor Functional Communication Profile. This evaluation is carried out on patients with aphasia by a certified speech pathologist upon admission and again at discharge. The scoring is done by giving the percentage of the over-all reduction of language modalities. Changes in communication ability are recorded for final scoring on the test profile.

DESCRIPTION OF PATIENTS IN THE STUDY

Patients were admitted to the Burke Rehabilitation Center from general hospitals of the greater metropolitan area of New York and Westchester County. Testing was done in weekly intervals until discharge. Six months after discharge data collection was initiated. Data obtained from the first 50 patients were evaluated to provide preliminary results. Of the 50 patients, 23 were right and 27 were left hemiplegic, secondary to cerebral infarction. There were 31 males and 19 females with an average age of 64 years; 8 patients had some degree of aphasia. The average length of stay in the Burke Rehabilitation Center was 57.8 days.

INITIAL RESULTS

Preliminary analysis of test data revealed that all patients in this study showed an improvement of motility as shown by the motility index, but the changes were small. Impaired motility was found on both the involved and uninvolved sides and improvement was observed to an almost equal degree on the involved as well as the uninvolved sides. Similar changes were found in strength measurements. Sensory changes have not yet been analyzed.

In groups with differing therapeutic exercise programs the fractional improvement of motility was almost identical. It was postulated that these specialized therapeutic exercises should improve motility. However, this appears not to be the case. The relative disproportionate improvement of the self-care status appears not to be related to the employment of the specialized therapeutic exercises as defined in this study. This has long been suspected by Diller and other observers.

CONCLUSION

A newly developed, automated statistical analysis program is currently in use and further data on the test results will be forthcoming.

A method of obtaining a profile expressed in numbers for the patient with stroke has been described. The nucleus of this profile is the quantitative assessment of motility defects within a quantitative, clinical, neurological test battery. The main objective of these efforts was to evaluate therapeutic measures in stroke rehabilitation. Preliminary analysis of some of the collected data on 50 patients showed that the employment of special therapeutic exercises ("patterning," etc.) had no influence on the motility of patients with stroke.

The motility test battery is now also used to assess changes of motility of patients with Parkinson's disease during a therapeutic trial with L-dopa.

SECTION V

Objective Behavioral Assessment in Diagnosis and Prediction

PRESENTATION 14

Manfred J. Meier

The purposes of this presentation are threefold: (1) to provide an overview of that portion of the neuropsychological literature which has some relevance for the assessment of behavioral outcomes in cerebrovascular disease by means of objective psychological methods, (2) to integrate relevant aspects of that literature into a preliminary description and interpretation of selected psychological test results for a series of patients with acute cerebrovascular symptomotology in Minnesota and in Japan, and (3) to formulate some suggestions and recommendations for future research into the behavioral consequences of cerebrovascular disease.

This examination of the role of objective behavioral methods in the assessment of cognitive deficits associated with cerebrovascular disease will necessarily emphasize research findings derived from patient populations exhibiting unequivocal clinical indications of an acute cerebrovascular episode. Definition of the relevant research domain in such a manner does not seem arbitrary when consideration is given to the fact that extensive atherosclerotic changes have been shown to be present in many older individuals in the absence of structural neuronal changes or gross neurological and other behavioral sequelae (Martin, Whisnant, and Sayre, 1960; Poser *et al.*, 1964; Millikan, 1967). The absence of such changes is entirely consistent with current knowledge of the hemodynamics of blood flow and the establishment of collateral circulation in cerebrovascular occlusive disease (Toole and Patel, 1967). Although subclinical atherosclerotic changes could conceivably be detected by means of behavioral assessment techniques, there is no evidence in man of measurable behavioral changes occurring independently of clinical neurological changes or as antecedent indications of an oncoming cerebrovascular episode. Thus, the little available data which may bear upon the question of behavioral correlates of cerebrovascular disease appear to be limited to the behavioral deficits resulting from acute cerebral infarction and ischemic attacks.

Since most neuropsychological research has not dealt directly with the behavioral correlates of specific disease processes, a rich data base for evaluating the efficacy of objective behavioral methods in the assessment of cerebrovascular accidents is not available. However, some studies have included sizable numbers of patients with completed strokes as representatives of the heterogeneous patient population with cerebral involvement or of a clinically well-defined population of patients with clearly lateralized cerebral lesions. Since it would be beyond the scope of this paper to review in detail all the neuropsychological research which might be relevant to the assessment of the behavioral consequences of cerebrovascular episodes, only an overview of this literature will be provided.

OVERVIEW OF THE NEUROPSYCHOLOGICAL LITERATURE

This body of knowledge can be viewed as an outgrowth of three converging areas of research activity: (1) clinical studies directed toward the development of global tests for detecting diffuse cerebral involvement and test batteries for localizing focal cerebral lesions; (2) theoretically oriented research designed to yield more incisive information about brain function through the assessment of the effects of focal neurosurgical ablations and of lesions in more selected populations such as patients with penetrating missile wounds; and (3) studies aimed specifically at elucidating the behavioral outcomes of cerebrovascular disease processes. All three domains appear to have relatively characteristic classes of methods and research emphasis, the third being less cohesive as a group effort and more uneven in research quality and sophistication.

CLINICAL STUDIES

Much of the post-World War II neuropsychological effort was devoted to a search for a single general behavioral method for detecting cerebral lesions, whatever the nature or location of the lesion (Klebanoff, Singer, and Wilensky, 1954). The generally poor performance of the many tests designed for this purpose contributed to an increasing awareness of the multivariate determination of behavioral consequences of structural changes in the brain and to the development of more elaborate test batteries (Halstead, 1947; Reitan, 1955b). These batteries incorporated both psychological (cognitive, perceptual, perceptual-motor) and neurological (sensorimotor, sensory suppression) levels of analysis in their methodology. Reviews of the validation studies supporting the clinical application of these batteries are available elsewhere (Reitan, 1962; Wheeler, Burke, and Reitan, 1963; Wheeler and Reitan, 1963; Yates, 1966).

The efficacy of the Halstead-Reitan approach was perhaps best exemplified by Reitan (1964) in an effort to infer location (left anterior, left posterior, right anterior, right posterior), extent (focal, diffuse), and lesion category (cerebrovascular disease, tumor, trauma, multiple sclerosis). These inferences, based exclusively on test data, age, and education, were compared with independently derived neurological ratings for a selected series of patients for whom neurological criterion information along these clinical dimensions was available. Agreement levels were uniformly high for the focal versus diffuse classifications, for the laterality of lesions located posteriorly (but not anteriorly), and for identifying type of lesion, with the exception of extrinsic tumors which were more difficult to identify on the basis of Halstead-Reitan battery results. Reitan was careful to interpret these concordance data with restraint by emphasizing the complexity of behavioral outcomes and their relations to structural and disease process variables and by reasserting the difficulty experienced in specifying the characteristics of the psychological measurements which differentially influenced the inference-making process.

These difficulties were highlighted further by an analysis of the statistical relations of the Halstead battery, the Wechsler-Bellevue Test (Form I), and the Trail-Making Test to the lesion location and lesion type classifications. Of 192 possible intergroup (test-criterion) comparisons of the focal lesion groups, only 25 reached acceptable levels of statistical significance, the latter being limited to the tactual performance and finger-tapping tests of the Halstead battery. The direction of these lesion-deficit relations was generally in accord with expectation on the basis of well-known contralateral effects of focal cerebral involvement. Analysis of the 192 measures by lesion type revealed only 13 which reached statistically reliable intergroup differentiations; 10 of these reflected the selectively lower mean values of the intrinsic tumor group. In general, the results suggested that patients with tumors and cerebrovascular lesions performed at lower levels than did the patients with extrinsic tumors and head trauma, while anterior lesions could not be clearly differentiated from posterior lesions within the same hemisphere. Thus, the data provided no striking evidence of homogenity of test score pattern by lesion type.

The general conclusions which can be derived from the Reitan study include: (1) intraindividual score patterns may reveal strong empirical relations to clinical criteria of location and type of lesion, and (2) numerous uncontrolled determinants may have obscured behavioral differences associated with the cerebral dimensions. Reitan pointed out that more refined methodological and statistical approaches will be needed to evaluate the behavioral effects of cerebral lesions more precisely. It might be argued similarly that these same considerations apply to the development of clinical criterion classifications and estimates of neurological deficit utilized in the clinical setting. A priori, it would appear that some uncontrolled variables (1) may lie outside the boundaries of immediate surveillance and control in the clinical setting, (2) often confound one another even within the more exacting clinical criteria developed to date, and (3) intrude as much at the criterion level as in contributing to group overlap on behavioral measurements. These considerations seem inevitably to require an examination of the relations between behavioral measurements and the longitudinal as well as cross-sectional outcomes of neurological disease processes. The preliminary findings of such a study in the area of cerebrovascular disease will be presented later as the primary component of this paper.

STUDIES OF NEUROSURGICAL ABLATIONS AND TRAUMATIC LESIONS

A number of laboratories have been concerned only incidentally with clinical objectives and have emphasized the application of methods derived from experimental psychology. This experimental posture has involved the testing of hypotheses derived from theories of brain function in terms of postulated effects of focal cerebral lesions on perceptual, learning, cognitive, and personality functioning. These activities appear to have been stimulated by a multitude of interdisciplinary influences arising out of developments in neurophysiology, physiological psychology, classical neurology, and correlative neuroanatomy. Relevant reviews of work done in various laboratories are readily available for the behavioral effects of gunshot wounds (Teuber, 1955, 1959, 1962, 1964; Semmes *et al.*, 1960; Weinstein, 1962), frontal lobotomy (Mettler, 1949; Crown, 1951; Sheer, 1956; Smith, 1960; Willett, 1961), frontal lobectomy (Milner, 1964), temporal lobectomy (Milner, 1954, 1962), and subcortical involvement (Riklan and Levita, 1965; Meier and Story, 1967). Major general reviews which have attempted to integrate this vast array of findings, including the European work in neuropsychology and classical neurology, are also available (Meyer, 1957, 1960; Piercy, 1964; Luria, 1966).

Many of the objective behavioral methods and novel clinical assessment procedures which have grown out of these efforts have not been generally assimilated and applied by investigations of the behavioral consequences of cerebrovascular lesions. The rapid development of methods and existing data provide a relatively untapped reservoir of information for increasing the methodological and theoretical sophistication of future clinical investigations into relations between structural changes of the brain and alterations in behavior. As an example of such a methodological extension, an attempt will be made in the presentation of data below to show how a method designed to elicit new knowledge of the effects of unilateral temporal lobectomy on the ability to adapt to rotations of visual space was effectively applied to predict neurological outcomes in patients with acute cerebrovascular symptoms.

BEHAVIORAL ASSESSMENT AFTER CREBROVASCULAR ACCIDENT

Only a few studies which utilized objective behavioral measurements have been done with deliberate emphasis on the outcomes of completed stroke. By far the richest source of methods and findings immediately relevant to the assessment of the behavioral consequences of cerebrovascular disease involves the neuropsychological literature cited above. The bulk of this evidence stands in support of the laterality hypothesis of cerebral function, namely, that lesions of the left (or dominant) cerebral hemisphere produce verbal deficits while lesions of the right (or nondominant) hemisphere generate impairment of visuospatial and spatial-temporal organization and integration (Reitan, 1962). Confirmation of interhemispheric asymmetry in function, as measured by objective verbal and nonverbal tests, was explored by means of the Wechsler-Bellevue scales which sampled both these classes of function (Andersen, 1951; Reitan, 1955a; Fitzhugh, Fitzhugh, and Reitan, 1961). While the direction of the discrepancy between the verbal and performance scales was frequently observed to be consistent with the laterality hypothesis, numerous contradictory findings have failed to confirm the apparent sensitivity of the Wechsler-Bellevue test as a means of detecting or lateralizing focal cerebral lesions (Heilbrun, 1956; Smith, 1965, 1966; Meier and French, 1966a). Nevertheless, the research with this test has been instrumental in stimulating extensive investigation of behavioral impairment in clinical neurological populations and in prompting a search for more powerful verbal and visuospatial assessment methods to assess interhemispheric differentiation of function.

Only occasional investigations which have focused predominantly on clinically defined samples of cerebrovascular patients have appeared in the literature. Bauer and Becka (1954) compared small samples of patients with left and right cerebrovascular accidents on three measures of nonverbal abstraction ability and on measures of tactual recall, visual-motor form reproduction, pictorial-situational comprehension, and judgment. They reported no differences as predicted between aphasic and nonaphasic subgroups, classified by means of the Halstead-Wepman Aphasia Test, on any of the tasks utilized. Instead, a trend toward greater impairment of the underlying functions was observed in those patients with right hemisphere lesions. Incomplete descriptions of the test procedures, the bases for rating severity of neurological dysfunction (on which the subgroups were equated), and the criteria for separating the small samples involved into frontal and nonfrontal groups render the evaluation of their conclusions difficult. Their findings are perhaps significant for adding credence to the role of the minor hemisphere in the mediation of complex nonlanguage functions, a conclusion which had been arising out of a number of related psychometric (Andersen, 1951; Teuber, Battersby, and Bender, 1951; Reitan, 1955a) and clinical studies (Paterson and Zangwill, 1944; McFie, Piercy, and Zangwill, 1950).

Hague (1959) reported deficits in visuospatial organization as measured by the Grassi Block Substitution Test (1953) in a group of 15 patients with right cerebral involvement associated with cerebrovascular infarction. A similar deficit on the Block Design Subtest of the Wechsler Adult Intelligence Scale (WAIS) (Gruen, 1962) was interpreted to reflect generalized effects of cerebral dysfunction after cerebrovascular accident. The block design performance deficit was unrelated to lesion laterality and degree of motor and sensory deficit. A sex difference was also reported, with females scoring lower on a number of psychological test variables, including selected Rorschach variables, a perseveration test (Cattell, 1936), and the Verbal Comprehension Subtest of the WAIS. Absence of a relation between degree of cognitive deficit and of sensorimotor impairment was interpreted as evidence for a predating psychological aging process in the generation of stroke. Although it is plausible that prodromal variables with behavioral manifestations could predate the occurrence of stroke, the cross-sectional design and small samples utilized in this study would seem to limit seriously the relevance of the data to this conclusion.

A later investigation which focused upon a group with neurological diagnosis of cerebral thrombosis (Evans and Marmorston, 1963) is noteworthy for the large number (108) of stroke patients included in the primary sample. This sample was limited in range to a postacute outpatient group without aphasia and with good recovery. Analysis of the data involved a comparison of the performances of this group with those of 96 myocardial infarction patients on the Rorschach, Proverb Interpretations (Wells and Ruesch, 1945), Draw-a-Man (Goodenough, 1928), Bender Gestalt (Bender, 1938), Raven Colored Progressive Matrices (1958), and WAIS Digit Span and Vocabulary Tests (Wechsler, 1955). Data interpretation was limited by the authors' failure to analyze for laterality effects and relations of test performances to degree of neurological deficit. Instead, intergroup comparisons were run with the expected finding that the cerebrovascular group performed significantly poorer than the myocardial group on most of the measures analyzed.

Thus this study was directed toward the diagnostic efficiency of these tests for differentiating between two patient populations, a problem of marginal clinical or theoretical interest.

As indicated earlier, many cogent investigations of cerebral involvement have directly examined the relations between behavioral outcomes and clinical variables in cerebrovascular disease. Some of these studies, however, have included sizable subsamples of patients with definitive clinical indications of previous cerebrovascular occlusive disease characterized by focal neurological deficits implicating the left or right cerebral hemispheres. It was felt that citation and comment relating to these studies might more appropriately be integrated into the main body of this presentation, a preliminary account of some behavioral data collected on series of patients with acute cerebrovascular symptomatology in Minnesota and Japan, or into the section on the assessment of subtle behavioral deficits.

BEHAVIORAL ASSESSMENT OF ACUTE CEREBROVASCULAR EPISODES: THE MINNESOTA-KYUSHU INVESTIGATION

PURPOSE

In 1962, the Minnesota Center for Cerebrovascular Research embarked upon a multidisciplinary team effort to assess a wide range of clinical, physiological, pathological, biochemical, and behavioral correlates of cerebrovascular occlusive episodes. These studies have been primarily concerned with early diagnosis, evaluation of the natural course of the disease, and prediction of disease outcomes over short- and long-term follow-up.

SAMPLING AND METHODOLOGICAL CONSIDERATIONS

Only patients who fulfilled the following criteria were accepted for investigation: (1) symptoms consisting of sudden onset of hemiparesis, hemihypesthesia, visual field losses, or brain-stem dysfunction such as diplopia, vertigo, dysarthria, nausea, or vomiting; (2) symptom onset less than 1 month before admission; (3) apparent stabilization without gross indications of deterioration in clinical status; (4) exclusion of hemorrhagic strokes as defined by clear cerebrospinal fluid with normal cell count and no xanthochromia; (5) no serious acute medical complication such as pneumonia or myocardial infarction; and (6) low likelihood of an alternative diagnosis on clinical grounds.

Following admission and diagnosis at the Hennepin County General Hospital and the St. Paul Ramsey Hospital, the patients were sent to the University Hospitals where the evaluation and tests were carried out. These included a neuropsychological test battery, electroencephalography, four-vessel angiography, formal speech evaluation, genetic assay, blood lipid analysis, and blood coagulation studies. Studies were done during a 7- to 10-day period, after which the patient was returned to the referring hospital for continued care during the subacute period. Neurological status was monitored daily and a complete neurological study was done upon admission and on the day of discharge. The psychological test battery was done on the second day of the hospitalization period. These evaluations were repeated approximately 1 year later when the surviving patients were readmitted for follow-up. A replication of these studies was begun in 1963 on a collaborative basis by an investigative team at the Kyushu University Medical School, Fukuoka City, Japan, in an effort to obtain comparative data in the assessment of the natural history of stroke in the two cultural groups. This report will emphasize the findings with a battery of psychological tests, analyzed for the relations of selected tests scores to an assortment of criteria which incorporated ratings of clinical neurological status on admission and extent of neurological change over the immediate and long-term follow-up periods.

CLINICAL NEUROLOGICAL CRITERIA

On the basis of the neurological examination obtained on the day of admission to the University Hospitals, each patient was rated on each of three scales:

1. *Lesion laterality:* Predominantly left hemisphere; predominantly right hemisphere; not lateralizable
2. *Degree of involvement:* 0—no involvement; 1—mild involvement characterized by mild hemiparesis and/or sensory deficit, minimal or no dysphasia, and ability to walk without assistance; 2—severe involvement characterized by dense hemiparesis or hemiplegia or by hemianopsia or global aphasia superimposed upon less sensorimotor impairment.
3. *Bilaterality of dysfunction:* Classified as bilateral involvement if (1) focal neurological signs were present on ipsilateral side, (2) disturbance of consciousness was a clear-cut manifestation of the stroke, or (3) sustained dysarthria was present

These three rated variables were translated into a coding system to provide the following inferential classifications:

L_1: Left hemisphere, unilateral, mild
L_2: Left hemisphere, unilateral, severe
$L_1 > R$: Bilateral, left > right, mild

$L_2 > R$: Bilateral, left > right, severe
R_1: Right hemisphere, unilateral, mild
R_2: Right hemisphere, unilateral, severe
$R_1 > L$: Bilateral, right > left, mild
$R_2 > L$: Bilateral, right > left, severe
$L_1 = R_1$: Nonlateralizable, mild
$L_2 = R_2$: Nonlateralizable, severe
$L_0 = R_0$: Normal

Similarly, degree of change in neurological status was rated with the prevailing clinical neurological findings on admission serving as the base line. Degree of neurological change over the 7- to 10-day period of initial hospitalization (short-term criterion) and over approximately a 1-year follow-up period (long-term criterion) was rated along the following change of status scale:

D—Death

I—No significant change in neurological status, increased magnitude of symptoms, or new neurological deficits emerged

II—Significant improvement in neurological signs occurred but major residuals still present (e.g., patient with hemiplegia now able to walk; aphasia improved clinically to level of effective communication)

III—Improvement in neurological signs developed so that minimal or no residual deficits were present (equivocal or isolated findings such as hyperreflexia, a Babinski sign, subtle sensorimotor deficits)

A symptom-free age-equivalent group (IV) was added as a normal reference sample.

Interrater reliability of these clinical variables as measured by interrater agreement percentages across national samples for experienced clinical raters on the Minnesota and Kyushu teams varied from 83 to 100 per cent for a number of different interrater pairs and triads in the clinical classifications and from 77 to 100 per cent in the change of status ratings (Loewenson, 1963). Although multivariate in composition, these global ratings provided some means of organizing a large amount of information in the clinical neurological assessment and provided a somewhat more elaborate clinical criterion than that afforded by lesion laterality or disease grouping alone. It was felt that these ratings, however crude, were at least clinically relevant and sufficiently reliable to provide a first step in building more refined criteria against which to assess behavioral deficits associated with cerebrovascular occlusions.

NEUROPSYCHOLOGICAL TEST PROCEDURES

The battery of tests utilized in these studies was not intended to provide a comprehensive assay of the many adaptive functions which may undergo decline after cerebral infarction. The selection of tests was influenced by (1) restrictions imposed by the relatively acute or subacute status of the target sample, (2) the level of technical competence in psychological testing which was readily attainable by the Japanese team, (3) a priori considerations involving the behavioral effects of stroke, (4) promising findings with tests being explored in our laboratory in relation to the effects of temporal lobectomy, and (5) the extensive language function evaluations already being supplied by Schuell and her coworkers in the center program. Thus, assessment emphases of the psychological test battery were in a nonverbal direction, but not exclusively so, since some verbal test components were included. These, however, involved tests for which published norms were available for the Japanese population. Brief descriptions of the tests and the scores utilized in later analyses are as follows:

Wechsler Adult Intelligence Scale (WAIS). This well-known test is fully described elsewhere (Wechsler, 1955). Individual subtest scores were not considered sufficiently reliable for analysis with the smaller Japanese sample. For this reason, the component age-corrected Verbal and Performance IQ's and Full-Scale IQ's were analyzed. Analyses of deviation quotients based on combinations of subtests which have heavy factor loadings on the three major factors measured by the test (Tellegen and Briggs, 1967) are being done and will be presented elsewhere.

Trail-Making Test. Both parts of the Trail-Making Test (Reitan, 1958b) were demonstrated nonverbally with subsequent administration of number and alternating number-letter test sequences. Japanese script was used for the letters in Part B in testing the Kyushu sample. The number of errors and the total time in executing each sequence constituted the measure used in the analysis. Errors in test execution were called to the subject's attention and the next correct step in the sequence was given with a pointing response by the examiner. Maximum time limits of 300 and 500 seconds were set for Parts A and B, respectively. A nonverbal correction procedure was applied when the patient made an error. A maximum of three errors on Part A and five errors on Part B was allowed before discontinuing testing, in which case the maximum time score was arbitrarily assigned. A qualitative "failure" classification was recorded if the patient committed one or more errors with the two subtests treated independently.

Porteus Maze Test. The most recent revision of the test was utilized (Porteus, 1959). Follow-up assessment involved use of the Extension Series which was previously shown to eliminate practice effects and yield identical means and standard deviations as the Vineland Revision on retesting (Porteus, 1955). A minor modification in scoring was introduced to accommodate the generally lower level of functioning in stroke patients. Testing was begun at age 5 instead of 7. If the patient failed at ages 5 and 6, testing was discontinued and a test age of 4 was assigned. Computed in this manner, the assumption was made that ages 3 and 4 of the children's series would be passed if administered. This 4-year convention was applied, however, in order to minimize failure experience for the most severely impaired patients. The Test Age (TA) and Test Quotient (TQ) based on the 14-year norms were used as measures of performance.

Seguin-Goddard Formboard (FB). This task involves a 12- by 18-in. board with 10 indented spaces of differing geometric form. Correspondingly shaped blocks can be placed into these spaces with or without visual mediation. In this application the patient was allowed to see the board while placing the forms. Three such practice trials were given for each hand separately and for both hands together. Following these practice trials, the patient was blindfolded and instructed to place the forms with both hands. Inability to place the 10 forms into the board within 5 minutes while blindfolded was scored "fail." If the patient was unable to manipulate the forms with the involved arm, practice and blindfolded testing were done with the intact arm only. When the patient while blindfolded was able to manipulate and place the blocks with both arms, each arm was timed separately before testing with both arms.

Ballistic Arm Tapping (BT). The total number of alternating ballistic arm movements, across a 20-inch tapping board was recorded over 30-second trial time intervals. Each arm was tested twice in succession, right arm first. A stylus was used so that precise counts could be made from contacts with metallic plates anchored to each end of the board.

Two-Hand Coordination Test. With a stylus in each hand, this task required the patient to trace simultaneously a triangle on the left and a quadrangle on the right. These geometric forms were indented in channels which were bordered vertically by electroconductive surfaces. When either stylus touched the sides of channel, a counter and the contact or error clock of a two-channel electronic motion analyzer (Smith and Wehrkamp, 1951) was activated. When both hands were successfully tracing the forms a second clock, the travel or successful time clock, ran. Two tracing conditions were utilized. Initially, the patient was instructed to trace in a clockwise direction with both hands (right-

right) for five trials in which five trips around the forms constituted one trial. Following these trials, the patient was required to execute five trials by moving the left hand in a clockwise direction while moving the right hand in a counterclockwise direction (right-left). The number of errors, error time, and successful time were recorded for each trial.

Quantification of Handwriting (HW). The task involved writing a series of 10 figures-of-eight at maximum speed on electroconductive paper connected to the two-channel electronic motion analyzer. Contact and noncontact durations were summated across individual figure executions within a trial. Five trials were run under distributed practice conditions (1 minute rest between trials) and five under massed conditions (no rest). Therefore, a contact and noncontact duration was available for each trial. These data will be presented elsewhere.

Quantification of Gait (G). Similarly, contact and noncontact (stride) times were obtained for five walking trials under standard pacing and under fast pacing conditions. An 11-ft. grid was utilized for separate quantification of each leg under both conditions. Data will be presented elsewhere.

Visual Discrimination Test (VD). Twenty-four visual discrimination problems were devised in a multiple-choice format (Meier and French, 1965a). These consisted of fragmented concentric circle patterns which provided rotational or structural cues for discriminating the one differing pattern from the remaining three identical patterns. No attempt was made to manipulate difficulty level systematically. The dark stimuli on white background were presented in fixed sequence in a dark room on 35-mm. slides projected onto a screen placed 8 ft. from the seated patient. A card with numbered quadrants was used by the patient as an aid in locating the differing pattern on a matching basis. All 24 problems were presented in order for five testing trials, two at 16 seconds per problem exposure, two at 8 seconds exposure followed by another trial at 16 seconds per problem. Durations were controlled by a Kodak automatic slide projector which was equipped with a 4-in. f 3.5 lens and 500-watt projection lamp. Number of discrimination errors for each trial and exposure duration condition was recorded for analysis.

Visual Space Rotation Test (VSR). A fuller description of this test can be found elsewhere (Meier and French, 1966b). In this application, two dove prisms through which the patient could view thumb and forefinger in a 2-in. field were mounted in a tube. The task involved drawing an *X* in a .75-in. square on electroconductive paper in order under three conditions of visual-field rotation (90° to the right, 90° to the left, and

180° inversion). If the patient failed to complete the task within 5 minutes, a "fail" score was assigned to the rotation condition being tested and readaptation to the next condition of the three rotation conditions was attempted. If the patient was able to complete the task within 5 minutes at a given rotation condition, four additional trials were run and the trial contact and noncontact durations were recorded by means of electronic techniques of motion analysis. Thus the basic measure culled from the readaptation data was the number of rotation positions failed (maximum of 3; minimum of 0). In addition, quantitative separations of the total time for task execution into the contact and noncontact components were available for those patients who could perform the task within the time limits.

Televised Space Reversal and Inversion Test (TV-RI). These procedures were only recently added to the battery. They are discussed here because of their apparent sensitivity, reflected in early findings, for detecting focal cerebral lesions with mild or equivocal neurological manifestations (Meier, 1967). Closed-circuit television techniques were used to provide greater flexibility in the construction of tests for the assessment of readaptation to systematic modification of visual space (Smith and Smith, 1962). In this application reversal and inversion of the visual image on the monitor were introduced by means of special circuitry in the camera. The patient monitored his performance on the television screen while shielded visually from direct view of his performing hand. Order of initial hand used and testing condition were randomized from one patient to the next. The task involved placement of the 10 forms of the upright version of the Seguin-Goddard Formboard (Reitan, 1955b) into their respective recesses on the board with each hand under each of the following conditions: (1) direct visual confrontation; (2) shielded from the hand and board while monitoring performance on the television screen under standard orientation of the field; (3) shielded from direct view with reversal of the visual field; and (4) shielded with inversion of the field. The total time for the 10-form placement for each hand under each testing condition constituted the primary measure recorded. A number of measures could be derived from these basic measures, including the mean time per form placement, the mean differences between the hands, and various ratios.

Other Tests. In addition to the above tests, the battery has included the Bender Gestalt Test, a time sense test which was discontinued on the basis of low reliability, and the four parts of the Benton Visual Retention Test (1963), the results of which have not been analyzed as yet. The Minnesota Multiphasic Personality Inventory (Hathaway and McKinley, 1951) was also given.

RESULTS AND DISCUSSION

Preliminary data analyses have revolved around three foci of inquiry: (1) findings of the Minnesota-Kyushu comparative study, (2) prediction of short-term and long-term neurological outcome on the basis of selected tests in the Minnesota sample, and (3) analysis of subtle behavioral deficits by means of special visual and perceptual-motor tests. The particular tests utilized in each of these areas were related to such considerations as the accumulation of reportable data for a given test, the obviously greater relative validity of some tests, and the suitability of certain methods to one or more of these areas of inquiry.

PRELIMINARY FINDINGS OF THE MINNESOTA-KYUSHU COMPARATIVE STUDY

Although growing in breadth of coverage, the initial effort of the Kyushu group was limited to those tests in the battery which were reasonably well known in Japan, for which Japanese norms were available, or which were within the immediate technical capability of the Kyushu group. The early portion of the Kyushu series consisted mostly of patients who were seen 3 months or more after symptom onset (Meier and Okayama, 1966). The present analysis has been limited to those later patients who were tested less than 30 days after onset of symptoms in strict accord with the sampling criteria being utilized in Minnesota.

Wechsler Adult Intelligence Scale (WAIS). Table 1 summarizes the distribution statistics for the Minnesota and Kyushu samples for the Verbal, Performance, and Full-Scale IQ's (VIQ, PIQ, and FSIQ). These data are presented as a function of the laterality and degree of involvement classifications. It can be seen that the proportion of patients with milder neurological deficits is higher in the Kyushu sample, an outcome which has been found for the larger series from which these patients were derived. Neither sample exhibits the expected lower mean VIQ in the left cerebral hemisphere groups. Although aphasic and nonaphasic patients were included in these left hemisphere samples, no WAIS scores were used if the patient could not function at or above the lowest limits of the Verbal and Performance Subtests. Comparison of aphasic and nonaphasic patients will be done in conjunction with findings based on the aphasia battery used at the center (Schuell, 1965). Whether or not presence or kind of aphasia will be related to the VIQ-PIQ discrepancy, it seems reasonable to conclude that cerebral infarction of the left hemisphere does not produce gross discrepancies on the cor-

TABLE 1. Wechsler Adult Intelligence Scale Distributions of the Minnesota and Kyushu Samples

Clinical classification (N)		VIQ	PIQ	FSIQ
		Minnesota Sample		
Left—1	$\bar{X}$	95.69	95.25	95.63
(15)	s	11.19	10.69	10.26
Left—2	$\bar{X}$	86.00	81.73	83.31
(26)	s	17.43	15.34	16.54
Right—1	$\bar{X}$	92.83	89.42	90.92
(12)	s	12.76	13.06	11.68
Right—2	$\bar{X}$	88.98	76.19	82.64
(42)	s	13.27	17.01	13.58
Left total	$\bar{X}$	91.88	89.00	90.15
(41)	s	17.17	16.77	17.05
Right total	$\bar{X}$	89.83	79.13	84.48
(54)	s	13.14	17.03	13.52
Total—1	$\bar{X}$	97.96	96.19	97.07
(27)	s	12.57	13.11	12.08
Total—2	$\bar{X}$	87.84	78.31	82.90
(68)	s	14.94	16.50	14.66
		Kyushu Sample		
Left—1	$\bar{X}$	90.40	85.20	87.30
(10)	s	19.87	13.75	14.90
Left—2	$\bar{X}$	115.33	85.00	102.33
(3)	s	11.37	19.00	12.33
Right—1	$\bar{X}$	102.79	100.14	101.57
(14)	s	12.78	13.20	10.21
Right—2	$\bar{X}$	98.88	83.75	90.38
(8)	s	11.58	14.94	11.97
Left total	$\bar{X}$	96.15	85.15	90.77
(13)	s	20.91	14.22	15.34
Right total	$\bar{X}$	101.36	94.18	97.50
(22)	s	12.23	15.72	11.95
Total—1	$\bar{X}$	97.63	93.92	95.63
(24)	s	16.91	15.14	14.05
Total—2	$\bar{X}$	103.36	84.09	93.64
(11)	s	13.37	15.11	12.73

$\bar{X}$, mean; s, standard deviation.

responding expected WAIS data dimensions. Although the Japanese left hemisphere sample is still rather small (N = 13), WAIS deficits appear to involve declines in the PIQ more than in the VIQ ($t = 2.58$, 11df, $p < .05$, correlated means), a paradoxical outcome which suggests that reductions in visuospatial functioning may occur as a general effect of cerebral infarction in the Japanese.

The data for the right hemisphere groups are somewhat more consistent with expectation. The mean VIQ-PIQ discrepancy reaches about

10 points in the Minnesota sample ($t = 5.89$, 52df, $p < .001$, correlated means) and 7 points in the Kyushu sample ($t = 2.18$, 20df, $p < .05$, correlated means). Degree of neurological involvement is clearly associated with a relatively lower PIQ in both the Minnesota ($t = 6.03$, 66df, $p < .001$) and the Kyushu ($t = 2.38$, 9df, $p < .05$) samples among the severely involved patients. These reductions result largely from the PIQ declines of the more severely involved right hemisphere subgroups of each sample ($t = 5.89$, 40df, $p < .001$; $t = 2.75$, 6df, $p < .05$). Interestingly, the more severely involved Kyushu patients tested out at a higher FSIQ mean level ($t = 2.36$, 78df, $p < .05$, uncorrelated means). This was largely due to a lesser over-all level of decline shown by the right hemisphere subgroup in the Kyushu sample. Thus, there is a suggested interaction between laterality and severity of involvement, reflected in the larger relative PIQ decline in the more severely involved right hemisphere subgroup.

The most significant findings, perhaps, are the absence of a lower VIQ following left hemisphere infarction in both groups, the appearance of significant reductions in PIQ with right hemisphere involvement in both groups, and the generally higher FSIQ mean in the more neurologically involved Kyushu subsample. Absence of a selectively lower VIQ level in relation to the left hemisphere involvement in etiologically mixed focal lesion samples has been reported prevously when aphasics were omitted from the analyses (Heilbrun, 1956), and in a large series of brain tumor patients irrespective of the presence of dysphasic disturbances (Smith, 1965, 1966). Arrigoni and DeRenzi (1964), on the other hand, in a series of patients which included a large number with cerebrovascular accident, found a lower VIQ with the left-sided lesions but no lateral difference in the PIQ. With additional exceptions (Heilbrun, 1956; Arrigoni and DeRenzi, 1964; Smith, 1965, 1966), selectively greater visuospatial declines, as evidenced in PIQ changes, have been reported after right hemisphere involvement (Andersen, 1950, 1951; Reitan, 1955a; Fitzhugh, Fitzhugh, and Reitan, 1961), along with consistent lateralized differences in rank differences correlations between rank orders of subtest means (Matthews, Guertin, and Reitan, 1962; Matthews and Reitan, 1964). The issue, however, is complicated further by inconsistent reports for related visuospatial tests such as the Raven Progressive Matrices where (1) lower scores have been found for patients with left hemisphere lesions (Meyer and Jones, 1957; Arrigoni and DeRenzi, 1964); (2) no significant interhemisphere differences have emerged (Costa and Vaughan, 1962; Colonna and Faglioni, 1966); (3) lateralized deficits appeared only in the presence of constructional apraxia in which lower scores were associated with right hemisphere involvement (Piercy and Smyth, 1962); (4) aphasics were not differentiable from nonaphasics (DeRenzi and Faglioni, 1965); and (5) aphasics showed lower scores compared with nonaphasics (Colonna and Faglioni, 1966).

In a recent study of a group of patients with cerebrovascular accident in which testing was done 3 months or more after symptom onset (Archibald, Wepman, and Jones, 1967a,b), more clear-cut visuospatial deficits were associated with right hemisphere involvement when comparisons on the Colored Progressive Matrices (Raven, 1958), the Perceptual Maze Test (Elithorn *et al.*, 1964), and the Grassi Block Design Test (1953) were made to left hemisphere patients who could comprehend the instructions. When nonaphasic left hemisphere patients were compared with right hemisphere patients who committed no errors on certain classes of items on the Language Modalities Test for Aphasia (Wepman and Jones, 1961), superiority of the left hemisphere group was observed only for the Elithorn mazes.

On balance, these inconsistent data, although generally favoring the laterality hypothesis, point up theoretical and methodological problems associated with the use of psychometric devices in neuropsychological research, including the assessment of cerebrovascular disease.

First, it is obvious that laterality does not operate as a unitary dimension in the determination of group differences on verbal and visuospatial tests. It is likely that this variable is potentially confoundable with many other conditions which affect performance on global tests such as the degree and kind of dysphasic and dyspraxic disturbance; general cognitive effects; location, kind, and extent of cerebral involvement; time since symptom onset; individual differences in the organization of cerebral function; systemic influences affecting the establishment of collateral circulation after acute infarction; visual field defects; nature and extent of sensorimotor impairment; premorbid level of function; personality factors in the reaction to illness; and even cultural factors, as this investigation will attempt to show. Many of these conditions have not been tightly controlled in neuropsychological studies so that the inconsistent findings for the laterality dimension for these more global psychometric methods should come as no surprise.

Second, the critical measures used in the search for lateral differences in cerebral function, by virtue of their varied sensitivity to these numerous determinants and of their complex factorial structure, are perhaps too global for isolating such differences. This contention is further supported by the relative insensitivity of the Wechsler-Bellevue and WAIS to static atrophic lesions in the anterior temporal lobe, and to the long-term effects of unilateral temporal lobectomy, where only a reduction on the Picture Arrangement Subtest has been reported to persist (Meier and French, 1966a).

TABLE 2. Trail-Making Test Error and Time Score Distributions of the Minnesota and Kyushu Samples

Clinical classification (N)		Errors A	Time A	Errors B	Time B
		Minnesota Sample			
Left—1	X̄	0.38	105.63	1.94	209.69
(16)	s	1.02	62.48	2.26	152.25
Left—2	X̄	1.19	202.25	4.16	370.84
(32)	s	1.40	98.05	1.59	182.58
Right—1	X̄	0.08	135.23	3.31	238.92
(13)	s	0.28	79.25	1.89	161.20
Right—2	X̄	1.00	185.18	3.50	371.78
(40)	s	1.01	93.35	1.96	163.57
Left total	X̄	0.92	169.96	3.42	317.13
(48)	s	1.33	98.49	2.10	187.83
Right total	X̄	0.77	174.81	3.45	339.19
(53)	s	1.25	91.96	1.93	171.45
Total—1	X̄	0.24	118.90	2.55	222.79
(29)	s	0.78	70.76	2.18	154.18
Total—2	X̄	1.08	192.71	3.79	371.36
(72)	s	1.37	95.16	1.82	171.03
		Kyushu Sample			
Left—1	X̄	0.82	161.54	2.09	209.09
(11)	s	1.40	94.30	2.39	178.06
Left—2	X̄	0.60	149.50	2.00	266.80
(4)	s	1.50	113.04	2.89	206.71
Right—1	X̄	0.43	141.07	1.79	273.64
(14)	s	0.85	80.33	2.29	161.48
Right—2	X̄	2.00	239.83	3.67	423.67
(6)	s	1.55	93.25	2.07	118.46
Left total	X̄	0.80	158.33	2.87	301.67
(15)	s	1.37	95.50	1.50	179.44
Right total	X̄	0.90	170.70	2.35	318.65
(20)	s	1.29	94.12	2.35	162.81
Total—1	X̄	0.60	150.08	1.02	280.88
(25)	s	1.12	85.49	2.29	165.54
Total—2	X̄	1.50	203.70	3.20	387.60
(10)	s	1.58	106.15	2.35	155.58

X̄, mean; s, standard deviation.

Trail-Making Test. The means and standard deviations for the Minnesota and Kyushu samples can be found in Table 2. No differences as a function of lesion laterality are present. Severity of neurological involvement appears to be operating as a main effect on the error and time scores of Parts A and B with the comparisons between the degree 1 and 2 subgroups of the Minnesota sample reaching the .01 level of confidence or better. The Kyushu error and time score differences between the severity subgroups are statistically significant for Part B only,

TABLE 3. Porteus Maze Test TA and TQ Distributions of the Minnesota and Kyushu Samples

Clinical classification (N)		TA	TQ/14
	Minnesota Sample		
Left—1	$\bar{X}$	11.66	89.81
(16)	s	2.15	16.57
Left—2	$\bar{X}$	7.70	59.20
(25)	s	2.00	15.37
Right—1	$\bar{X}$	10.68	82.27
(11)	s	3.36	25.91
Right—2	$\bar{X}$	8.77	67.25
(32)	s	3.59	27.66
Left total	$\bar{X}$	9.43	71.15
(41)	s	2.82	19.32
Right total	$\bar{X}$	9.26	71.09
(43)	s	3.59	27.73
Total—1	$\bar{X}$	11.26	86.74
(27)	s	2.70	20.75
Total—2	$\bar{X}$	8.30	63.72
(57)	s	3.02	23.26
	Kyushu Sample		
Left—1	$\bar{X}$	14.00	107.58
(12)	s	2.39	18.38
Left—2	$\bar{X}$	15.00	115.33
(3)	s	1.50	11.49
Right—1	$\bar{X}$	13.42	101.54
(13)	s	3.56	27.08
Right—2	$\bar{X}$	10.00	76.80
(5)	s	4.54	22.35
Left total	$\bar{X}$	14.20	109.13
(15)	s	2.24	17.17
Right total	$\bar{X}$	12.47	94.67
(18)	s	4.04	29.72
Total—1	$\bar{X}$	13.70	104.44
(25)	s	3.01	23.05
Total—2	$\bar{X}$	11.88	91.25
(8)	s	4.37	31.73

$\bar{X}$, mean; s, standard deviation.

but larger sample sizes will probably confirm a difference on Part A inasmuch as these approach significance at this time. None of the differences between the Minnesota and Kyushu samples is significant so that performance appears to be similarly effected. These findings confirm previous reports (Reitan, 1958) of the sensitivity of this test to cerebral dysfunction generally but fail to support indications of differential impairment of the relative A-B time discrepancy which has been related

TABLE 4. Matching Variable Distributions of the Minnesota and Kyushu Subsamples

National source	Sex	Laterality	Degree		Age	Education	FSIQ
Minnesota	16 M 7 F	10 L 12 R 1 =	14—1 9—2	$\bar{X}$ s	59.00 8.33	9.09 2.54	92.26 10.60
Kyushu	17 M 6 F	12 L 10 R 1 =	14—1 9—2	$\bar{X}$ s	59.65 7.36	8.57 2.54	92.52 13.37

$\bar{X}$, mean; s, standard deviation.

to lesion laterality in an etiologically mixed sample of patients with focal cerebral lesions (Reitan and Tarshes, 1959).

Porteus Maze Test. The rather striking differences between the Minnesota and Kyushu samples in the over-all levels of performance on the Porteus Maze Test can be seen in Table 3. Firstly, laterality does not appear to be related to performance level in either sample. By contrast, TA means differ significantly when degree 1 and degree 2 subgroup comparisons are made within the left and right hemisphere subgroups of the Minnesota sample pointing up a direct relation between degree of neurological involvement and impairment in performance on the Porteus Maze Test ($t = 5.10$, 82df, $p < .001$). This relation seems less clear-cut in the Kyushu sample, where patients with predominantly right score insignificantly lower than patients with predominantly left cerebral involvement.

The most striking feature of these data is the over-all difference between the national samples where all subgroup comparison t-ratios are significant at the .05 level or better. In order to elucidate these differences further, a t-test for correlated means was computed on the basis of differences in Porteus TA between 23 patient pairs matched for age, education in years, lesion laterality, degree of neurological involvement, and WAIS FSIQ. Table 4 shows the matching variables distributions. Matched pair data for the Porteus TA can be found in Table 5. With pairs almost perfectly matched on each of these variables, the resulting TA differences continue to be highly significant ($p < .001$) with the Kyushu group scoring 3.54 TA years above the Minnesota group. The extent of this difference is further indicated by the level of subsample differentiability achieved by means of a cutting score of TA = 12 which correctly identifies the national origin of 78.3 per cent of the combined samples.

These considerable differences in Porteus Maze Test performances are subject to a number of interpretations. First, cross-cultural research

TABLE 5. Porteus Maze Test Comparisons for Matched Pairs

	WAIS FSIQ		Porteus TA		
Pairs	Minn.	Kyushu	Minn.	Kyushu	TA diff.
1	109	101	16.5	16.5	0.0
2	93	107	11.0	15.0	+4.0
3	98	106	13.5	17.0	+3.5
4	98	103	8.0	11.0	+3.0
5	101	107	14.0	16.0	+2.0
6	95	100	9.5	9.5	0.0
7	90	108	6.0	13.5	+7.5
8	110	108	11.0	16.5	+5.5
9	90	90	8.5	9.5	+1.0
10	83	83	9.0	13.5	+4.5
11	108	105	12.5	15.5	+3.0
12	93	89	10.0	12.5	+2.5
13	79	70	7.0	10.5	+3.5
14	96	95	10.5	17.0	+6.5
15	82	77	8.5	15.5	+7.0
16	92	88	5.0	11.0	+6.0
17	91	94	11.5	12.5	+1.0
18	67	60	4.0	4.0	0.0
19	72	73	9.0	15.5	+6.5
20	92	90	12.0	13.0	+1.0
21	98	99	7.0	13.5	+6.5
22	91	92	11.5	15.0	+3.5
23	94	83	9.0	12.5	+3.5
$\bar{X}$	92.26	92.52	9.76	13.30	+3.54
s	10.06	13.37	3.07	3.10	0.88

$t = 4.02$, 22df, $p < .001$

Cutting point (TA)			
≥ 12	4	17	(78.3%)
< 12	19	6	

$\bar{X}$, mean; s, standard deviation.

is always fraught with sampling problems, although the matching analysis would appear to have minimized the intrusion of such factors as much as possible within the framework of the study. Second, it is well known that the Japanese tend to score somewhat higher on this test than do other national groups (Porteus, 1933, 1959). These differences account for the relatively mild performance declines observed in the Kyushu sample after cerebral infarction. Thus, it seems reasonable to conclude that these differences may constitute a behavioral expression of population differences in the cerebral organization of the functions measured by the Porteus mazes. The implied differential cerebral organization of function conceivably could eventuate from multivariate influences involving cultural differences in the developmental facilitation of skills relevant to maze test performance or possibly even racial-genetic factors. Viewed as a possible greater resistance to functional decline after cerebral infarction in the Japanese, over-learning facilitated by differing cultural influences would seem the more reasonable alternative since intergroup differences have not been as strikingly evident on the other measures of cognitive functioning used in these analyses. In any case, the possibility that cultural conditions can serve to increase the resistance of certain functions to decline after structural neuronal changes have occurred is an intriguing implication of this comparative study, but may serve to complicate even more the establishment of generalization validity of behavioral devices in assessing the effects of focal cerebral lesions in man.

BEHAVIORAL PREDICTION OF NEUROLOGICAL OUTCOME

The evidence for complex multivariate determination of individual variation in psychological test performances associated with cerebral lesions has contributed to a more deliberate control and systematic manipulation of such variables as laterality, location, extent, and acuteness of cerebral lesions in recent investigations (Reitan, 1962). Although many variables are amenable to study by cross-sectional sampling of appropriate neurological populations, the temporal behavioral dynamics of neuropathological processes require prospective or longitudinal assessment strategies. Surgically introduced ablative lesions, usually superimposed upon a static epileptogenic neural substrate, have been investigated for their effects on the longitudinal course of cognitive functioning following prefrontal and temporal lobe ablations (Meyer, 1960; Meier and French, 1966a). Comparisons between etiologically heterogeneous neurological samples varying in time since symptom onset have been made (Fitzhugh, Fitzhugh, and Reitan, 1962), but clinically critical short-term behavioral changes following acute onset of neurological symptoms have not been elucidated.

Perhaps more than any other class of lesions encountered in the neurological setting, the thrombotic stroke provides a wide range of interpatient variability in the reversibility of neurological symptoms. Although maximal neurological losses occur in a fair proportion of cases, as much as 25 to 30 per cent of patients who show even profound paralysis may recover much or all of the lost functions in the days or weeks following onset of symptoms (Harris and Towler, 1955). The predictability of such changes from behavioral bases obtained early in the recovery period might reflect extent of reversible loss, provide incisive prognostic estimations, and illuminate some of the dynamics of infarction-induced cerebral lesions at the behavioral level of analysis.

TABLE 6. Psychological Test Score Distributions as a Function of Short-Term Neurological Change

Measure		Neurological change groups			
		I (N = 44)	II (N = 26)	III (N = 23)	IV (N = 58)
Age	Mean	68.11	61.54	65.13	68.71
	Sigma	7.70	12.09	8.13	6.61
WAIS FSIQ	Mean	73.16	85.81	97.30	111.09
	Sigma	15.63	17.96	11.82	11.50
Porteus TA	Mean	5.45	7.98	11.33	12.57
	Sigma	2.41	3.31	3.79	2.65
Ballistic tapping	Mean	29.85	48.38	77.72	87.13
(both arms)	Sigma	26.08	35.08	20.28	20.03
Visual Discrimination	Mean	17.40	15.32	12.35	8.61
(No. of errors)	Sigma	2.27	4.30	4.63	4.98
Trails A	0/0 Fail	75	27	13	3
Trails B	0/0 Fail	97	85	52	36
Formboard	0/0 Fail	93	65	39	3
Visual space rotation	3F	33	16	4	3
(Freq.—No. of positions fail)	2F	2	4	2	6
	1F	0	0	4	10
	0F	2	2	11	36

As a preliminary attempt to explore the potential validity of behavioral methods for predicting evolving changes in neurological status following acute onset of cerebrovascular symptomotology, various tests in our battery were analyzed for their relations to the criterion of rated neurological change over the initial period of hospitalization (Meier and Resch, 1967). Some behavioral test distribution data obtained on the second day of hospitalization, shown as a function of the short-term change classifications and the normal (IV) reference group, can be found in Table 6. The test measure means follow a constant intergroup ordering with the "no change" group (I) scoring at the lowest performance levels on each test. Progressively higher test mean and percentage pass values across groups are consistent with the inference that level of behavioral functioning on the second day of hospitalization varies linearly with rated change from the first to the final day of hospitalization.

From this broader battery of tests a subbattery was selected on the basis of apparent predictive validity, ease of administration and scoring, and brief total administrative time of approximately 1 hour. This battery included the Porteus Maze Test, the Trail-Making Test, the Seguin-Goddard Formboard, and the Visual Space Rotation Test.

Test predictors for maximizing group separations could be isolated by examination of inter- and intraindividual variation in test score in

TABLE 7. Percentage of Short-Term Change Groups Showing Differentiating Signs of Group I

Predictor	Group I	II	III	IV
Porteus TA <6	61	11	4	0
Fail trail making: A + B	73	27	13	0
Fail formboard	93	61	39	3
Two or more signs	77	19	8	0

each neurological change group. As shown in Table 7, separation of Group I from Groups II and III was relatively well achieved by determining the percentage of patients within each group that fulfilled at least two of the following test criteria: Porteus TA <6, failure on Parts A and B of the Trail-Making Test, and failure on the Seguin-Goddard Formboard. Application of a two-sign convention led to classifying 77 per cent of Group I patients correctly while misclassifying 19 per cent and 8 per cent of Groups II and III, respectively.

Groups I and II were separated from Group III by empirical determination of the cutting points with a low frequency of fulfillment in Group III which simultaneously maximized identification of Groups I and II. Table 8 shows the percentage of patients in each group which fulfilled the following criteria: Porteus TA equal to or less than 8; failure on two or more positions of the VSR Test; failure on Part B on the Trail-Making Test and on the Seguin-Goddary Formboard. Application of a combined two-sign convention maximized Group III separation from Groups I and II with only 19, 9, and 5 per cent misclassification of Groups III, II, and I, respectively.

Since predictive efficiency of these test predictors over longer periods of time is of greater clinical significance, their efficacy was assessed

TABLE 8. Percentage of Short-Term Change Groups Showing Differentiating Signs of Group III

Predictor	Group I	II	III	IV
Porteus TA ≤8	84	65	21	9
Fail trail-making B and formboard	91	62	30	0
Visual space rotation fail 2 or more signs	95	91	29	16
Two or more signs	95	91	19	6

TABLE 9. Percentage of Long-Term Change Groups Showing Differentiating Signs of Group I

Predictor	Group D	Group I	Group II	Group III
Porteus TA <6	50	63	25	5
Fail trail-making: A + B	68	67	25	5
Fail formboard	86	85	63	26
Two or more signs	61	67	25	0

against rated neurological change from the first day of initial admission to neurological status at a follow-up interval of 1 year or more. The percentages of each long-term follow-up group which showed the most characteristic test signs of Group I, the "no change" group, on the short-term criterion can be seen in Table 9. The decreased and Group I long-term criterion patients exhibit the test predictors of Group I considerably more frequently than do Groups II or III. Similarly, in Table 10, test predictors which differentiated Groups I and II from Group III on the short-term change criterion, when applied to group identified in terms of long-term neurological change, continue to maintain reasonably high predictive utility.

In order to estimate the relative efficiency of such behavioral predictors it would seem most relevant to compare the efficacy of the tests with "hit rates" based upon (1) the sample base rate for neurological outcome and (2) the initial degree of rated neurological involvement. Meaningfulness of the sample base rate as a future predictor would, of course, depend upon the representativeness of this sample to those which might be collected in other similar hospital settings. Sample base rate as defined here simply involves the percentage of patients who in fact are classified in each of the four long-term follow-up groups.

TABLE 10. Percentage of Long-Term Change Groups Showing Differentiating Signs of Group III

Predictor	Group D	Group I	Group II	Group III
Porteus TA ≤8	71	85	50	5
Fail trail-making B and formboard	82	85	50	21
Visual space rotation, fail 2 or more	89	93	75	16
Two or more signs	89	85	50	10

TABLE 11. Correct Hit Percentages for Broader Differentiations of Combined Groups

Predictor	Combined group percentages					
	D + I	Hit	II + III	D + I + II	Hit	III
Sample base rate	67 →	67	← 33	77 →	77	← 23
Initial severity						
1	18 ↘		↙ 55	22 ↘		↙ 57
		64			72	
2	82 ↗		↖ 45	78 ↗		↖ 43
Group I test signs	65 →	75	← 7	59 →	68	← 0
Group III test signs	87 →	84	← 22	83 →	84	← 10

Predictions based on degree of neurological involvement might have immediate generality since they are as independent of sampling considerations as are behavior test scores.

The four change groups were subdivided in two ways for assessing the predictive efficiency of each class of predictors. The D and I groups should be differentiable from Groups II and III on the basis of the Group I test signs. Similarly, the D group was added to Groups I and II to determine the efficacy of the predictors in separating these groups from Group III. Table 11 shows the hit percentages of the various predictors. The hit percentages are the percentages of these combined groups which could be accurately differentiated from each other on the basis of a particular class of predictors. Thus, for the sample base rate, if it is predicted that all the patients will show D or I outcomes, the percentage of correct hits would be 67 and for predicting that each patient will fall into Group D, I, or II the percentage of correct hits is 77. Those percentages simply reflect the fact that 67 per cent of the total group outcome was D or I, while 77 per cent was D, I, or II. If it is predicted that initial severity 1 will be associated with improvement (II or III) and severity 2 with no change (D or I), over-all predictive accuracy on the basis of initial degree of neurological involvement is 64 per cent. Similarly, in predicting eventual status in Groups D, I, and II rather than in Group III, 72 per cent of the outcomes are predictable on the basis of initial severity. Both Group I and III test signs yield higher hit percentages (75 and 84, respectively, against the short-term neurological change criterion) than either the sample base rate or degree of initial neurological involvement. The separation of Group III from the combined D, I, and II groups is maximized at 84 per cent predictive accuracy with application of the Group III behavioral predictors. Group I test predictors are less effective than the base rate and degree of neurological involvement variables in making this differentiation. Among the classes of predictors being considered, the Group III test predictors consistently yield the higher hit rates for predicting the long-term outcomes as rated.

It should be emphasized that this began as a clinical exercise to provide some rather rough estimations of the kinds of changes the clinical neurologist considers relevant in his usual assessment of the patient. We are merely using these results as a basis for future exploration of neurological change and the development of behavior predictors in cerebrovascular disease. In this direction, Ettinger and I are conducting a study at the Hennepin County General Hospital of fresh admissions for acute cerebrovascular symptomology. Sequentially frequent monitoring, both psychological and neurological, might provide measures of value for prediction and for the development of a more objective and reliable criterion of neurological change. Although these data show that change can be reliably rated in a global manner within 30 days and again 1 year after symptom onset, it is likely that the first 2 weeks may be the most critical in the emergence of change. In a clinical study of hemiplegia due to cerebral infarction (Twitchell, 1951), major neurological changes were documented in the 6- to 36-day interval of the symptomatic course, some observable changes appearing as early as 48 hours after symptom onset. Our continued investigation of such outcomes, and their early predictability in the natural course of stroke, has been prompted by the apparent potential predictive utility of behavioral tests and the opportunity provided by the stroke patient to explore the plasticity of the nervous system in accommodating to cerebral infarction. In addition, such careful monitoring of neurological and psychological change might lead to the development of more sensitive behavioral methods for detecting early central nervous system changes in cerebrovascular disease and subclinical residuals of small focal infarcts, static atrophic lesions, and "silent area" involvement—lesions which have been relatively difficult to diagnose with objective neurological signs or psychometric devices.

EARLY DIAGNOSIS AND SUBTLE BEHAVIORAL DEFICITS

These considerations lead us into some critical issues regarding the role of behavioral assessment in the early diagnosis or early detection of cerebrovascular disease. Diagnosis after symptom onset in acute cerebral infarction would hardly seem to require special assessment strategies since only 3 patients in our entire series were misdiagnosed (Balow, Alter, and Resch, 1966). This is in general agreement with other clinical studies of cerebrovascular accident (Carter, 1964; Silverstein and Hollin, 1965). Objective behavioral measurement of individual differences among patients after the establishment of the clinical diagnosis can be expected to yield information of value for assessing nature and extent of cognitive impairment and for predicting neurological outcome after completed strokes. This level of contribution appears feasible with relatively brief and easily administered test batteries which do not require elaborate instrumentation or technical resources. More comprehensive batteries can be utilized if needed, although the effort expenditure would not appear to be justified for general diagnostic purposes. Therefore, future diagnostically oriented behavioral research might more profitably be directed toward the evaluation of behavioral precursors of developing cerebrovascular changes and the subtler deficits associated with elusive clinical events such as transient ischemic accidents and small infarcts in association cortex or white matter which produce mild, equivocal, or no objective neurological deficits.

PREMORBID DETECTION

There are a number of considerations which complicate the development of effective behavioral research strategies in the early detection and measured anticipation of oncoming cerebrovascular accidents. As was stated earlier, it has been clearly shown that extensive plaque formation is present in many older individuals without related neuronal changes and that structural concomitants of cerebrovascular disease are dependent upon the systemic dynamics of blood flow and the utilization of the available collateral circulation. Extent of visualizable plaque formation, derived from four-vessel angiography, does not correlate highly with the clinical symptomotology in completed stroke (Amplatz, 1966). Stenoses of hemodynamic significance are often absent so that reliable criteria of the neuropathological correlates of cerebrovascular disease may be available only at autopsy, preceding which many other intervening neuropathological events can have confounded the correlatable vessel and structural changes in the brain.

The outlook for finding behavioral predictions of oncoming cerebrovascular accidents would seem rather poor on these grounds alone. An earlier recommendation (Benton, 1961) to do a major prospective study was based upon the retrospectively reported incidence of behavioral "lapses" in patients who subsequently developed cerebrovascular accidents. No major longitudinal studies have been done. However, we have replicated our clinical studies, excluding angiography, on about 150 symptom-free volunteers over age 60 and have followed these for a year or more. The 1 patient who has had a cerebrovascular accident to date showed no conspicuous prodromes on any measure in the protocol. It is estimated that 1,000 cases would need to be followed to yield 15 to 20 completed strokes per year. The formidable and expensive nature of such an undertaking probably accounts for the lack of effort in this area of research.

Mention should be made of a modest behavioral assessment program now underway in Hisayama, Japan. All residents past the age of 40 in this community of 14,000 are being evaluated and followed with some of the shorter psychometric tests of our battery including the Porteus mazes and the Trail-Making Test. As the validity of the most incisive brief tests being utilized in our laboratory becomes established it is planned to selectively apply them in the Hisayama study. The problems associated with developing neuropathological and neurophysiological criteria of structurally significant cerebrovascular disease and with the low prevalence rate of cerebrovascular accidents will no doubt reduce the likelihood of obtaining the yield being sought, namely, valid prediction of an oncoming cerebrovascular accident or ischemic attack on the basis of behavioral methods. Nevertheless, the Hisayama project may provide the only available context for doing a meaningful prospective behavioral study.

ASSESSMENT OF SUBTLE DEFICITS

As shown earlier, where conspicuous behavioral deficits are present, qualitative indicators of the patient's test performance can contribute to the evaluation of behavioral status and the prediction of neurological outcome. If the validity of such measures is maintained after cross-validation and further refinement of techniques and outcome criteria on new stroke patients, monitored over the days immediately following admission, then the more obvious deficients reflected in these indicators should be fairly readily assessed. Screening for conspicuous sensorimotor and perceptual cognitive deficits in neurological settings has been shown to be efficiently attainable with rather gross techniques (Costa *et al.*, 1963). The subtle behavioral deficits observed in patients with cerebrovascular accident and with mild or equivocal neurological residual deficits, however, may require more elaborate, time-consuming, and complicated behavioral testing devices. Prevalent and potentially powerful instruments are available in the growing literature cited earlier on the behavioral effects of focal atrophic lesions, lobectomies introduced in the treatment of neocortical seizure disorders, and gunshot wounds. Analogously, methodological applications in our laboratory aimed at eliciting subtle deficits in cerebrovascular disease were in part derived from our recent interest in complex visually guided behavior and perceptual motor functioning in relation to static focal cerebral and subcortical lesions. Where relevant, background data will be reviewed and

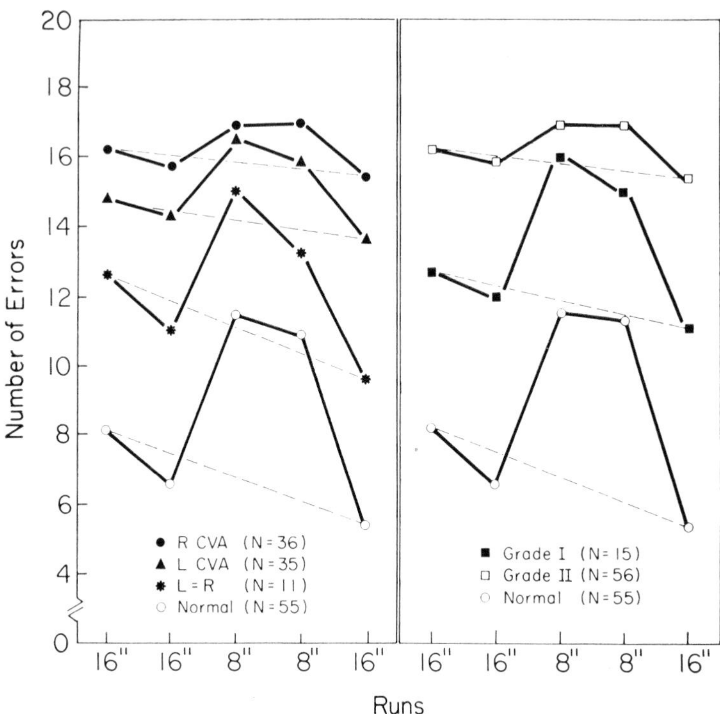

FIGURE 1. Visual discrimination error means as a function of laterality and degree of neurological involvement.

selected findings in our series will be presented for a number of these tests.

Visual Discrimination. The discriminability of fragmented circle patterns was shown to be significantly more impaired after right compared with left temporal lobectomy in psychomotor epileptics (Meier and French, 1965a). Figure 1 shows the mean error scores for subgroups of left and right cerebrovascular accident, basilar vertebral insufficiency (L = R), and age-equivalent normal controls. The completed stroke sample mean scores analyzed in terms of degree of neurological involvement are also presented. All patient groups clearly differ from the normal group on this task, while the completed stroke patients differ from the insufficiency subgroup. Although the group with right cerebrovascular accident exhibits somewhat higher error scores than the group with left cerebrovascular accident, these differences are not statistically significant. An interaction between laterality and degree of neurological involvement is evident from analyses (not shown here) which reveal higher error means in the right—1 compared with the left—1 hemisphere group with very little overlap between the groups. Thus, the test shows

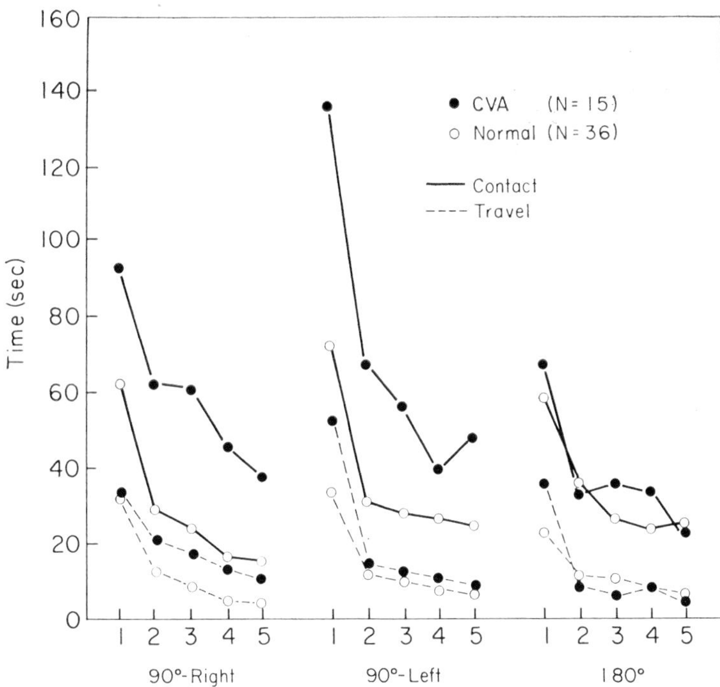

FIGURE 2. Contact and travel durations in readaptation to visual space rotation.

promise for differentiating laterally among the less involved patients after completed stroke.

Visual Space Rotation Test. Previous research in our laboratory (Meier and French, 1966b) failed to elicit differences between left and right temporal lobectomized patients on a more elaborate version of this task. However, patients with extratemporal spike foci generated longer contact times in the two-channel temporal quantifications obtained under a number of differing conditions of rotation. This suggested a mass action basis in the cerebral cortex for deficits on this task. It will be recalled that the majority of patients who showed considerable short- and long-term improvement was able to readapt to each of three rotation conditions utilized. Combined, these data suggest that subtle defects resulting from mild alterations in cerebral status might be manifested by elongation of one or both of the quantifiable temporal components of task execution in such patients (Meier and Resch, 1966). Figure 2 shows the comparison between this select patient group and age-equivalent normals on five trial blocks for each condition of rotation. The cerebrovascular accident subgroup exhibits significantly longer contact time means at 90° right and 90° left of standard. Since a minority of older normals have some difficulty (see Table 6) with this task and quantitative deficits are observed even in the patients with recovery potential, it was felt that this kind of method might be highly sensitive to subtle changes in cerebral status.

This is consistent with other recent findings in relation to a block rotation task showing that patients with cerebral lesions of varying etiology, especially with cerebrovascular occlusion, have difficulty in reproducing stationary block designs in rotated fashion (Satz, 1966a). Similarly perceptual-motor deficits have been observed in older hemiplegics in the ability to judge the visual vertical and horizontal (Birch *et al.*, 1960a), judge the medial plane (Birch *et al.*, 1960b), and analyze complex visual patterns (Birch and Belmont, 1964).

Space Reversal and Inversion Test. The above findings served as a basis for developing a modification of the Visual Space Rotation Test which seemed more suited to elderly patients. The method also combines the neurological and psychological approaches by assessing the effects of alterations of visuoperceptual input conditions upon motor readaptation on the side contralateral to the lesion. The assumption was made that such manipulations would exaggerate or amplify subtle contralateral perceptual-motor deficits. A number of patients with mild, equivocal, or no objective neurological deficits (Meier, 1967) consisting of our follow-up patients with mild cerebrovascular accidents and a group with relatively small neurosurgically removed gliomas detected in the prefrontal and temporal regions before major proliferation, were tested under conditions outlined earlier.

Figure 3 shows the mean time per block placement for the left (N = 12) and right (N = 16) hemisphere groups as well as an age-equivalent (N = 20) normal control group. Only small differences in mean time magnitude appear on the contralateral side with form placement under direct confrontation. Even under standard visual field conditions the mean time per block placement shows increased elongation on the contralateral side in each laterality group, while the normal group times increase bilaterally without reaching the ipsilateral durations of the lesion groups. These contralaterally expressed exaggerations of mean time increase in a progressively upward direction under reversal and inversion of visual space.

The directional differences in these findings can perhaps be described more clearly by examining the average difference between the hands as a function of lesion laterality and testing condition. Figure 4 shows that these differences increase in magnitude, differ in algebraic sign across testing conditions in the left and right hemisphere groups, and remain unchanged at or around zero in the normal group. Since the

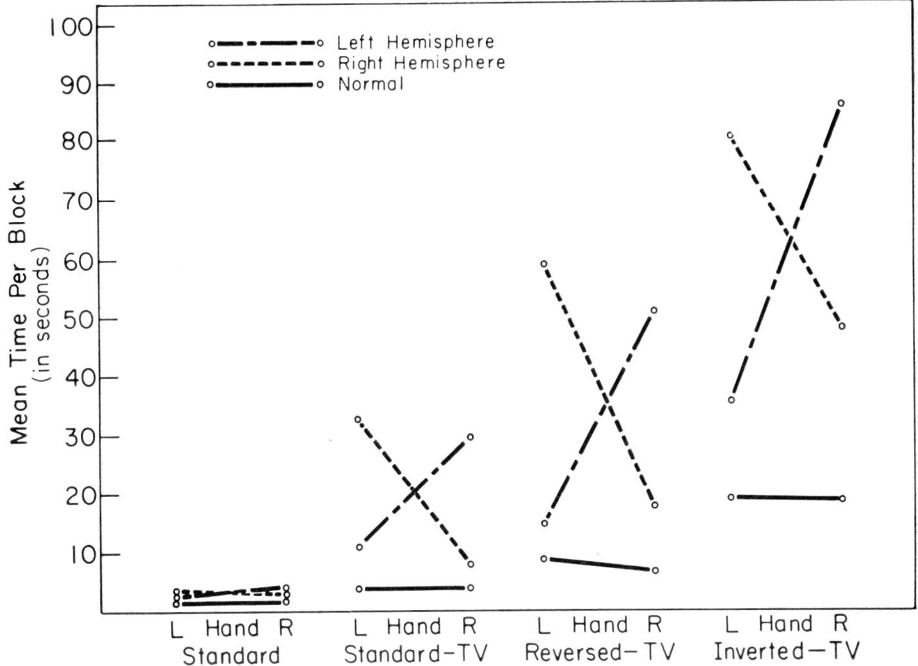

FIGURE 3. Mean time per block placement on the Seguin-Goddard Formboard Test under standard, reversed, and inverted visual space conditions.

variances (not shown here) around the patient group means also increase as the testing conditions become more difficult, the distribution-free or nonparameric median test was applied to evaluate differences between the patient groups and between each patient group and the normal group. Overlap between groups was relatively minimal on the R-L difference measures so that highly significant chi-square values ($p < .001$) emerged from the median test applications. Utilizing a cutting score of —4.5 on the R-L measure, 84 per cent of the laterality groups could be differentiated from each other and from the normal control group. By contrast, the WAIS VIQ-PIQ discrepancy (10 points or greater with sign predicting lesion laterality) correctly lateralized only 61 per cent of the lesions. Lesion laterality inferred from the WAIS was at chance level for the left, but well above chance for the right, hemisphere lesions.

Since the present samples are as yet limited in size and since these methods will need to be validated on patients tested before neurological diagnostic decisions have been made, the results of this study are insufficient to evaluate the utility of these measures for detecting subtle behavioral deficits. Observation of sizable and frequently profound quantitative increase in the time scores of the hand contralateral to the lesion

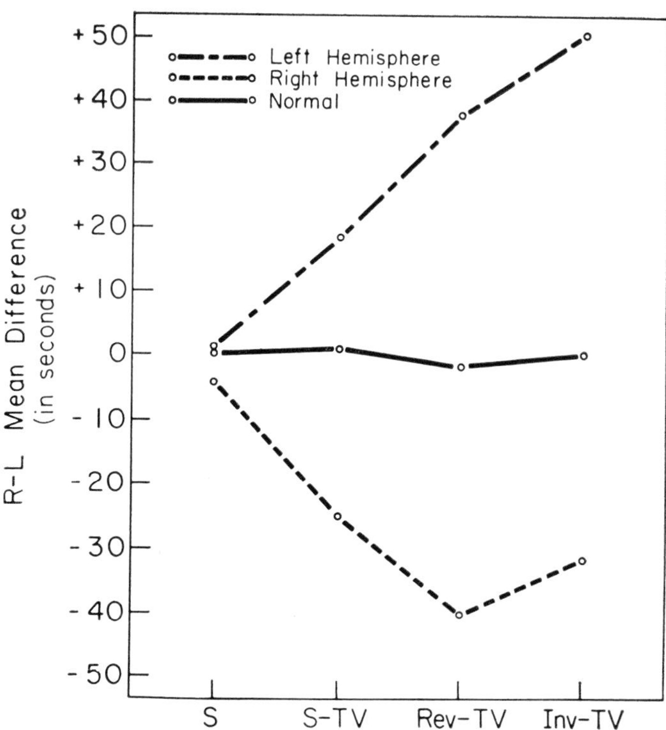

FIGURE 4. Mean difference between hands in block placement under standard, reversed, and inverted visual space conditions.

in patients with equivocal or no pyramidal tract findings would appear to warrant further exploration of these methods for developing behavioral indices of subtle deficits in cerebrovascular and other lesions affecting the cortex.

Related methods of potentially high yield in eliciting residual deficits in cerebral disease can be found in studies of reaction time and focal cerebral lesions. Benton and Joynt (1959) reported greater slowing of the contralateral hand in a choice reaction-time task with lesions of the right, but not as clearly with lesions of the left, cerebral hemisphere. Brain-damaged patients generally showed slowed reaction times bilaterally as compared with normals. Similarly deficits in discrimination of short temporal duration (Van Allen, Benton, and Gordon, 1966), intensity estimation of successively presented auditory stimuli (Birch, Belmont, and Karp, 1967), and cross-modal reaction time (Benton *et al.*, 1962) in brain-damaged samples with sizable cerebrovascular accident subgroups have been demonstrated. Thus, vigilance tests may be more sensitive than global intellectual tests in detecting cerebral lesions (De Renzi and Faglioni, 1965) although patients with functional disorders,

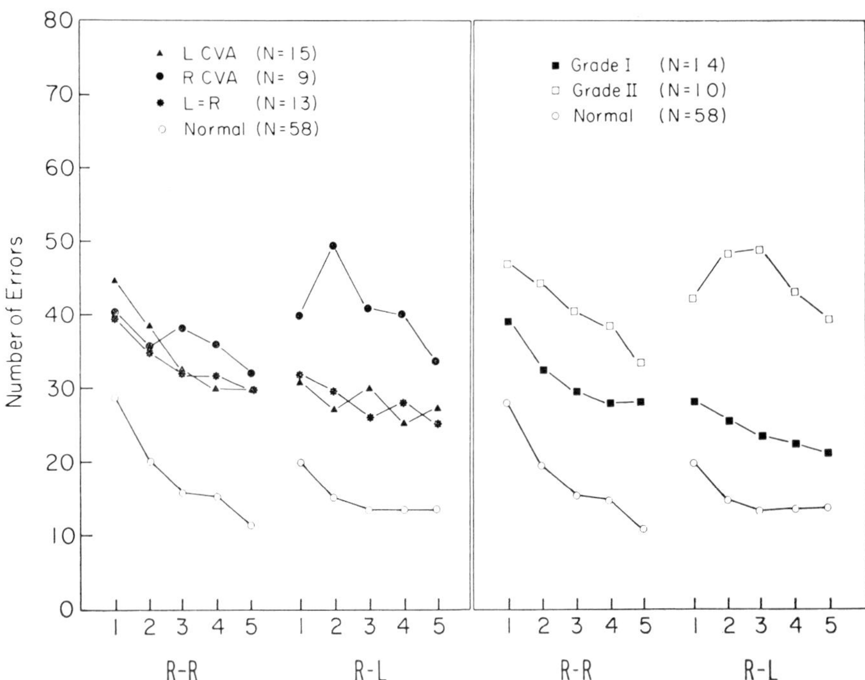

FIGURE 5. Mean number of errors in two-hand coordination as a function of lesion laterality, degree of involvement, and direction of hand movement.

especially schizophrenics, tend to exhibit impairment of vigilance (Benton, Jentsch, and Wahler, 1959, 1960).

Two-Hand Coordination Test. Relatively few patients in our series have been able to perform this task. Therefore, we discontinued its use in the battery. Reexamination of the data on those patients who could meet the requirements of the test is suggestive of some potential of this kind of measurement for assessing subtle deficits associated with cerebrovascular lesions.

Figure 5 shows the mean number of errors for 24 patients with completed stroke (15 left and 9 right), 13 with a diagnosis of vertebral basilar artery insufficiency, and 58 age-equivalent normal controls. Additional data of the completed strokes, divided in terms of degree of neurological involvement, are also presented. All three cerebrovascular disease samples show higher error means when both hands are engaged in coordinating the styli in a clockwise direction (R-R). When the hands are then moved for five trials in opposite directions (R-L), the patients with right hemisphere damage exhibit a rather marked negative transfer effect; yet all three groups continue to differ from the normals. The milder completed stroke subsample (I) shows lower error mean levels than the severely involved group (II). Again, subtle deficits appear to be involved. We have now reintroduced a modification of this test using triangular forms and measuring simultaneously yet independently the temporal components of error and successful performance of each hand.

The above applications constitute only a few of the procedures which can be devised with closed-circuit television and electronic motion analytic techniques. The construction of such behavioral test procedures is obviously almost limitless. For example, we are currently exploring pegboard task performances, form tracing, and pointing tasks with each hand under reversal, inversion, and rotation conditions. Such methods would seem potentially capable of providing rapid assessment of samples of older individuals for screening purposes in prospective research and for the efficient detection of subtle residuals and monitoring behavioral course after cerebrovascular occlusive episodes and other kinds of focal cerebral involvement. Obviously, much research remains yet to be done. This overview of the ongoing clinical neuropsychological research would seem to indicate that objective behavioral approaches promise to provide a meaningful adjunct to traditional clinical methods in the assessment of cerebrovascular disease.

PRESENTATION 15

Ralph M. Reitan

Meier began his paper with a rationale for delimitation of his investigation to patient samples who exhibited unequivocal clinical indications of an acute cerebrovascular episode. His rationale cited the prior finding that human beings may have sustained extensive atherosclerotic changes in the absence of neuronal alterations or gross neurological or behavioral deficits. He went on to indicate that no evidence has been presented to the effect that measurable behavioral changes occur independently of clinical neurological deficits and therefore even the "little available data" on behavioral correlates of cerebrovascular disease appear to be limited to patients with acute cerebral infarction and ischemic attacks. As is well known, however, many patients have diffuse (or multifocal) cerebrovascular disease without gross neurological or behavioral changes even though their symptoms are sufficient to bring about neurological evaluation and diagnosis. This group is undoubtedly of considerable clinical significance. For example, such a group is reported by Marshall and Shaw (1959) to have an even higher mortality rate during a 4- to 9-year follow-up period than groups with acute cerebral infarcts. Omission of such a group, therefore, would appear to represent a significant deficiency in assessing behavioral correlates of cerebrovascular disease generally considered. Because of the need for such information, and in order to round out the information available in this workshop, a group of patients with clinical evidence of diffuse cerebrovascular disease was included in a study that I shall report later in this discussion.

The criteria for acceptance of patients in the Minnesota Center for Cerebrovascular Research relate specifically to selection of patients with focal occlusive cerebrovascular disease rather than patients with diffuse cerebrovascular disease or cerebral hemorrhage. Thus, it is important to note that the patient groups reported by Meier represent focal occlusive cerebrovascular disease rather than cerebrovascular disease more generally. The clinical neurological criteria, described by Meier, represent a significant advance in terms of development of criterion information against which to evaluate psychological test results. As pointed out by Meier, these clinical variables are relatively crude and difficult to define, and result only in global ratings. However, the efforts reported by Meier along these lines represent a significant advance in consideration of what previously has been done in this area of investigation. Definition of criteria and standardization of procedure are absolutely imperative as a basis for assessing changes in patients over time. Without this kind of approach no reliable criteria would be available with respect to improvement shown by certain patients.

A great number of factors may represent possible bases for explanation of different results reported by various investigations, as Meier makes abundantly clear. Undoubtedly problems of examiner influence, epidemiological composition of samples, and many other influences will gradually have to be sorted out in order for conclusions in this area to reach a point of increased precision. Meier has knowledgeably identified many of the possible factors that may be of significance in this respect, including external variables as well as consideration of the nature of the psychological measures themselves. This type of rationale may be extended even further with respect to the results Meier obtained using the Trail-Making Test. While Meier failed to confirm the previous report of Reitan and Tarshes (1959), it should be noted that the differential performance on Parts A and B of the Trail-Making Test, as related to lateraliation of cerebral damage, can be tested only by using a standard score transformation of the data. The absolute time differences between the two parts of the test appear to vary in significance depending upon their magnitude. Thus, a raw-score analysis is relatively unrevealing, whereas an analysis of comparative difficulty controlled through transformation to a normal probability distribution makes the effect more clear. Thus, in addition to the various factors that Meier mentioned, mathematical data transformation and specialized statistical methods may be necessary for demonstration of certain effects regardless of their degree of validity.

Finally, the evidence Meier presented which suggests the definite possibility of the influence of cultural conditions with respect to differential ability levels as well as to degree of deficit following cerebral infarcts has a number of interesting implications. First, we again learn the lesson of caution with respect to generalization of research results. Second, the relation of premorbid ability structure to psychological deficit following cerebral damage is emphasized. Finally, the necessity for detailed individual studies in order to define the behavioral concomitants of particular types of cerebral lesions, since they may differ from one culture to another, is indicated. Only gradually have we been learning that a whole host of variables influences the psychological effects of lateralized and localized cerebral lesions, including individual differences in biological characteristics of brain function from one individual to another, individual differences in premorbid psychological ability structure, and, differences that may even characterize entire cultural groups.

Meier's results concerned with prediction of neurological outcome on the basis of psychological test performance stand as a most important pioneering effort in this area. A considerable number of studies have been reported in the literature that ostensibly are concerned with this type of problem. However, these studies are retrospective in nature and merely identify factors that are *associated with*, rather than *predict*, eventual outcome. When reported in this manner their predictive potential remains unknown. However, Meier has in fact determined the predictive efficiency, at least in a preliminary manner, of various types of indices with respect to the short-term and longer-term neurological outcome. The results appear promising and, in addition to providing some information with respect to psychological and neurological recovery, may, as Meier indicated, provide additional insight into the nature of psychological changes associated with cerebrovascular disease.

The contribution of behavioral assessment to early diagnosis or to early detection of cerebrovascular disease is scarcely answered, as implied by Meier, by the number of patients in his series with acute cerebral infarction who were misdiagnosed. The clinical neuropsychological problem frequently is not diagnosing acute cerebral infarct but rather evaluating psychological deficits in patients with possible evidence of early cerebrovascular degenerative changes. Much emphasis has been directed traditionally toward the use of behavioral and psychological test assessments for purposes of neurological diagnosis. The intention is scarcely to replace traditional neurological diagnostic methods or to imply that such methods are deficient in achieving their intended purpose, but rather to study the relations between results obtained from at least partially different domains. In this way psychological and neurological findings can be interrelated as a basis for developing an improved understanding of brain-behavior relations. However, without demonstrating the existing relation between psychological and neurological data (and this can often best be accomplished by predicting one from the other), a groundwork has not been established for using patients with neurological deficits as a basis for studying brain-behavior relations. The point is not to use a comprehensive psychological test battery for neurological diagnostic purposes, but rather to evaluate behavioral functions dependent upon the integrity of the cerebral hemispheres.

In his discussion of the assessment of subtle deficits associated with cerebrovascular disease, Meier observed that such deficits, in association with mild or equivocal neurological findings, may require fairly elaborate, time-consuming, and complicated behavioral testing devices. Since he has focused his study not on patients with mild or equivocal neurological findings, but rather on patients with behavioral deficits associated with completed strokes, this speculation of Meier is only of passing interest. As will be demonstrated later in this discussion by presentation of empirical results, our findings indicate that patients who show at most mild and in most instances equivocal or noncontributory neurological signs and symptoms are about equally impaired in a general sense as patients who have suffered lateralized cerebrovascular lesions. As mentioned previously, our results indicate that this group clearly needs detailed and special study in its own right. In fact, the presence or absence of specific deficits on physical neurological examination seems relatively unrelated to the *degree* of impairment on a broad battery of psychological tests demonstrated to be significantly dependent upon the integrity of the cerebral hemispheres. In his closing remarks Meier presented preliminary data on a number of examining procedures that promise useful results in assessment of subtle deficits in patients with cerebrovascular disease. The approaches outlined are interesting experimentally and are potentially important in clinical assessments. The preliminary results obtained by Meier, however, are not surprising in consideration of results we have obtained in our laboratory. As Meier indicated, much research remains to be done in exploring subtle deficits, but objective behavioral methods of measurement appear to have considerable promise in contributing to a fuller understanding of the neuropsychology of cerebrovascular disease.

The charge to Meier and to the discussants has been admirably fulfilled in most respects by the paper he presented. Many of the questions to which he was able to address his presentation were beyond the limits of the current work of my own laboratory. Fortunately, however, we find ourselves in a position to make certain additions to the presentation. We have had an opportunity to study small groups of patients not only with lateralized cerebrovascular lesions but also with diffuse or generalized cerebrovascular disease, both with and without significant deficits on physical neurological examination. Also, we have had the opportunity to perform preliminary explorations with regard to the question whether cerebrovascular disease produces a distinctive pattern of behavioral loss as contrasted with cerebral neoplasms and traumatic lesions of the cerebral hemisphere.

Our purpose in the study presently to be reported was to obtain comparative information on patients with lateralized cerebrovascular lesions and patients with diffuse cerebrovascular disease. Four groups of subjects were used. The first group consisted of 20 patients with focal vascular lesions of the left cerebral hemisphere; the second group of 20 patients with right cerebrovascular lesions; the third of 26 patients in whom diagnostic evidence indicated bilateral or generalized cerebrovascular disease; the fourth of 26 persons who had no past or present evidence of cerebral disease or damage. This last group served essentially as a normal reference group with respect to brain function. In each of the groups with lateralized cerebrovascular lesions, the onset for each patient was sudden, and diagnostic evidence supported the conclusion that one cerebral hemisphere or the other was maximally involved.

While clinical neurological criteria for composition of groups always present a problem, the degree of error is clearly less for some categories than others. The category of diffuse, generalized, or multifocal cerebrovascular disease is one of the more difficult in terms of generally valid inferences. Nevertheless, the category undoubtedly is an important one and must be studied, even though eventual improvements in criterion information or group composition may bring about modifications of resulting conclusions. Thus, in the recognition that scientific progress must be expected to come about as a series of increasingly precise approximations, a group with clinical diagnoses of diffuse or bilateral cerebral vascular disease was composed for comparison with the other groups. In addition, however, a fairly detailed description of the signs and symptoms demonstrated by members of this group will be presented to facilitate evaluation by the reader and comparison with results obtained by others.

The presenting complaints of patients judged to have generalized or diffuse cerebrovascular disease were multiple in all instances, although in some cases the complaints related to only two or three types of difficulties whereas in others they covered a wide range. In nearly all instances both somatic complaints and symptoms relating to higher-level psychological deficits were mentioned. Headaches (N = 9 or 35 per cent) and episodes of dizziness (N = 8 or 31 per cent) were among the most common somatic complaints, although 7 patients (27 per cent) complained of tingling, numbness, or some degree of weakness of one or both upper extremities. Less common were complaints relating to visual, olfactory, or gustatory loss. Several patients complained of burning sensations of the extremities, roaring sounds in the ears, clumsiness in movement, a burning sensation of the eyes, easy fatigability, or general nervousness. Very few patients did not include in their presenting complaints difficulties relating to higher-level psychological functions. Most commonly cited was memory loss (N = 10 or 38 per cent), but patients also complained of word-finding or speech difficulty (N = 6 or 23 per cent), crying spells or other indications of emotional lability (N = 6 or 23 per cent), episodes of confusion (N = 3 or 12 per cent), depressive episodes (N = 2 or 8 per cent), and deterioration of handwriting (N = 1 or 4 per cent). Neurological evaluations were done on each patient, including all procedures necessary for reaching a differential diagnosis. The physical neurological examination was reported to yield entirely normal results in 9 (or 35 per cent) of the 26 subjects. The

TABLE 12. Diagnosis in 26 Patients With Diffuse or Bilateral Cerebral Vascular Disease

Diagnosis	N
Diffuse cerebral arteriosclerosis	18
Hypertensive encephalopathy	5
Bilateral internal carotid artery disease	2
Basilar artery insufficiency due to arteriosclerosis	1

remaining 17 subjects, in the main, had minimal or isolated signs or deficits of equivocal diagnostic significance. Thus, the entire group may be viewed as one in which positive findings from the physical neurological examination were relatively minimal, although data analyses were done to compare the 9 subjects with entirely normal results and the 17 with minimal or isolated findings. The minimal findings reported on physical neurological examination included such disturbances as slow or somewhat slurred speech, mild tremor of the hands, some possible weakness of the upper extremities, and possible diminution of light touch and vibratory sensation. A few patients, however, had more definite findings. For example, 2 patients were judged to have definite mild hemiparesis and 2 additional patients were found to have quadrantic homonymous visual field defects. In the main, however, findings on the physical neurological examination did not reveal any striking or profound deficits. Electroencephalography was done on 23 of the 26 patients, with findings reported as being entirely normal in 8 (35 per cent) of the subjects; 3 subjects were reported to have focal slow waves, but in the remaining 15 patients the findings were reported as representing dysrhythmia, which was mild in nature in 13 of the 15 patients. Contrast studies were done on 13 of the 26 patients, including 6 pneumoencephalograms, 2 ventriculograms, and 12 angiograms. In no instance did the results indicate the presence of a focal cerebral lesion. The diagnoses for the 26 patients in this group, all based on evaluations performed during one or more hospitalizations, are shown in Table 12. It should be mentioned that a number of associated diagnoses were present. These included 3 instances of diabetes mellitus, 2 of myocardial ischemic disease, 2 of arteriosclerotic heart disease, and 1 each of hypertensive cardiovascular disease, depressive reaction, movement disorder, cervical osteoarthritis, and right radial nerve palsy. While certain of these conditions may have been associated with cerebrovascular disease, the diagnosis for cerebrovascular disease required additional findings for substantiation in every instance. At the present time, 4 of the patients are known to be dead. Although an autopsy was performed on only 1 of these patients, all were reported to have died of cardiovascular or cerebrovascular disorders.

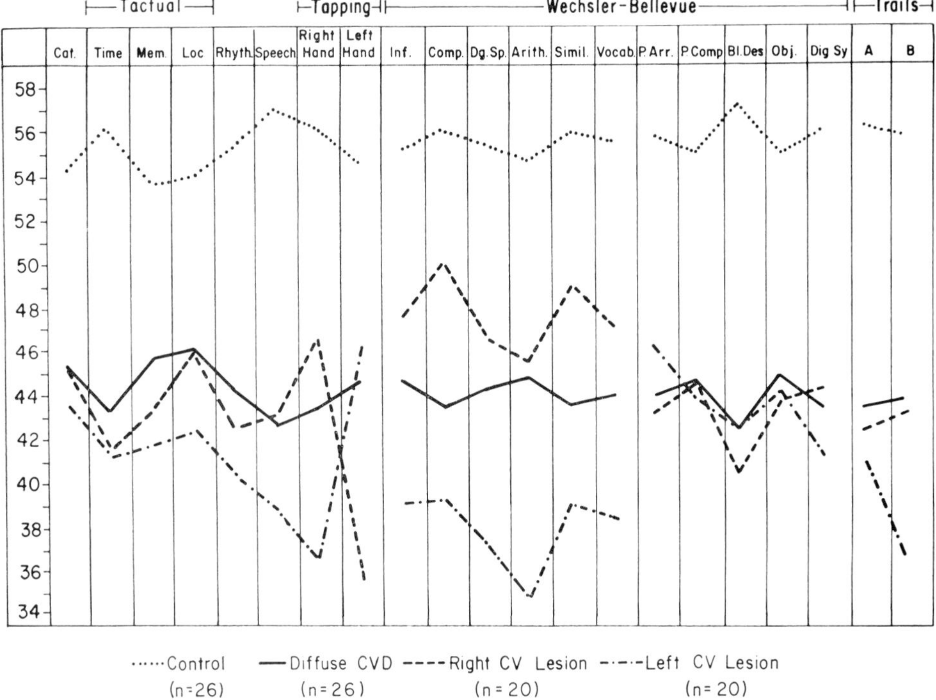

FIGURE 6. Performances of controls and patients with cerebrovascular disease.

The results of comparisons of the three groups with cerebrovascular disease and the control group are presented in Figure 6. Proceeding from the left to the right side of the figure are listed tests from Halstead's neuropsychological battery, the Wechsler-Bellevue Scale, and the Trail-Making Test. The vertical axis represents a normalized T-score scale having a mean of 50 and a standard deviation of 10. The transformation from raw scores was effected by combining the 26 patients without cerebral lesions and the 26 patients with diffuse or generalized cerebral involvement. On the basis of transformations from raw to T-scores for these two groups, scores were assigned to the patients with right or left cerebrovascular lesions.

It is apparent that the group without cerebral damage performed considerably better on all measures than did any of the groups with evidence of cerebrovascular disease. Statistical analyses of the data indicated that for every possible comparison of individual means between the control group and any group with cerebrovascular disease, the difference was significant in favor of the group without cerebral damage. Thus, we can conclude that in terms of level of performance any of the groups with cerebrovascular disease was generally impaired, with the generality being represented by the fact that impairment occurred on every measure used in the study. The three groups with cerebrovascular disease were not significantly different on measures from Halstead's battery, except for the lateralization effect on finger-tapping speed. Thus, Halstead's tests consistently reflected impairment of all three groups that was approximately equivalent in degree. On the Wechsler-Bellevue Scale, however, an effect was present that related to laterality of cerebral damage. While the group with diffuse or bilateral cerebral damage tended to have almost identical levels on the Verbal and Performance Subtests, the group with right cerebral lesions had lower mean scores on each of the Performance Subtests than on any of the Verbal Subtests. The reverse situation was true for the group with left cerebral lesions: The mean scores for the Verbal Subtests were lower than the mean scores for the Performance Subtests. This effect, which was noted as being variable from one study to another by Meier, may well require transformation of raw scores to normalized distributions to demonstrate itself with clarity. However, again, our results confirm our previous findings. It should be noted in the instance of the data in this particular study that it is difficult to obtain significant intergroup differences on these variables. Statistical comparisons of the groups are complicated by what appear to be sampling artifacts. While the differences in the *Verbal* Subtests for groups with right and left cerebral lesions were consistently significant in this particular comparison, the effect occurred obviously because the group with right cerebral damage tended to have somewhat higher total scores on the Wechsler-Bellevue Scale than the group with left cerebral damage. This sampling deviation tended to maximize the differences between the Verbal Subtests and minimize the difference between the Performance Subtests, even though the comparative relationships of Verbal and Performance Subtest scores within the groups were consistent with lateralization of cerebral damage. The Trail-Making Test demonstrated deficits in all groups with cerebral lesions, although significant differences between the groups with cerebrovascular disease were not present.

Meier raised a question about the possible degree of psychological deficit that might be shown by patients with minimal, if any, findings on physical neurological examination. We had an opportunity to explore this question in preliminary form by subdividing the group with diffuse cerebrovascular disease into 9 patients who had entirely negative neurological findings and 17 patients with minimal positive findings. Figure 7 presents the results for these two groups together with the results for the total group from which they were drawn. The results are plotted on exactly the same axes as were used in Figure 6. It is apparent that differences between these two groups are minimal. No statistically sig-

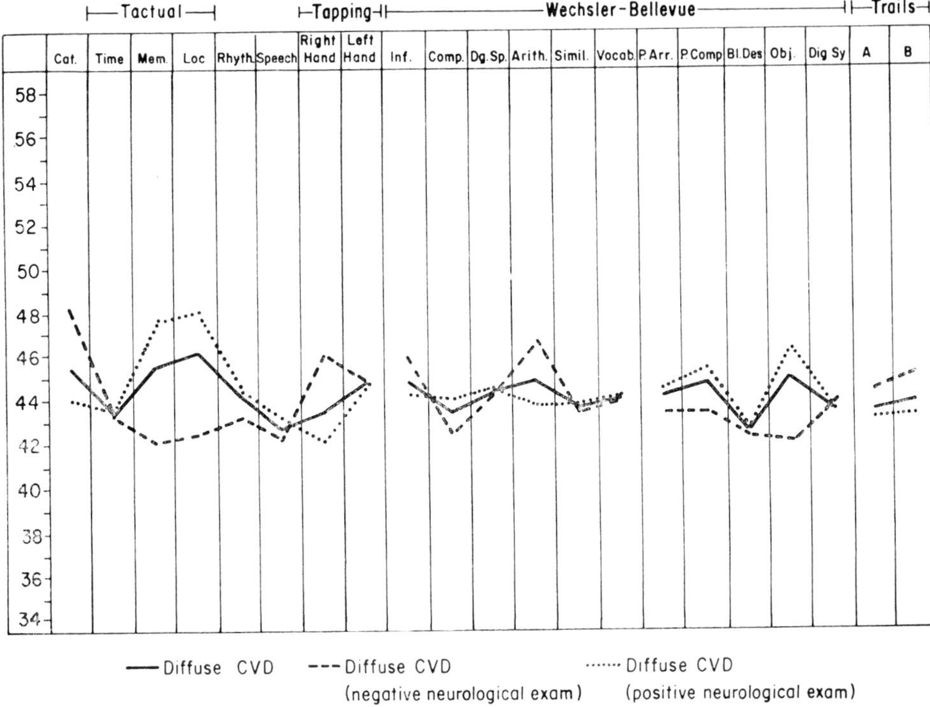

FIGURE 7. Performances of patients with cerebrovascular disease with and without positive neurological findings.

nificant differences were present. It would appear that subjects with cerebrovascular disease, even in the presence of normal neurological examinations, still demonstrate significant impairment of abilities as measured by objective psychological tests.

The remaining item in the specific charge to the author and discussants with respect to the topic under consideration concerned whether cerebrovascular disease produces a distinctive pattern of behavioral loss. From a procedural point of view alone, this question is immensely difficult to answer, in spite of the fact that variations in type of lesions represent one of the principal neurological characteristics of cerebral damage. Most investigations, as noted by Meier, have used heterogeneous groups of subjects with varied types of lesions and therefore have not been relevant to this neurological dimension. A few studies have restricted themselves to examination of subjects with a single type of lesion, but these, in turn, have been limited at least to some extent in their generality. A fundamental problem which limits progress in this area relates to the time-consuming process of composing groups of subjects within appropriate neurological categories for study. Nevertheless, a comparative evaluation of the possible differential effects of various types of cerebral lesions would seem imperative in the development of further understanding in this area.

At present we have underway at Indiana University Medical Center an organized program of investigation aimed toward effecting a comparison of the psychological correlates of cerebrovascular, neoplastic, and traumatic lesions. While this study is presently ongoing and final results are not yet available, the comparisons have been based on triads of subjects matched for color, sex, age, and education. In addition, each of the groups of subjects, selected according to type of lesion, was further subdivided into three groups in accordance with lateralization or diffuseness of cerebral damage. Thus, the research plan called for a total of nine groups (right, left, and diffuse cerebral involvement within categories of cerebrovascular, cerebral neoplastic, and cerebral traumatic damage). A tremendous number of patients in total was required in order to hold constant the variables of color, sex, age, and education, and only 15 subjects could be identified for each of the nine subgroups.

The results, in preliminary form, indicate that patients with cerebrovascular or neoplastic disease were somewhat more seriously impaired in terms of level of performance than patients with traumatic injuries, although a substantial degree of overlap occurred between groups. Measures related to motor speed and motor strength of the upper extremities (finger-tapping speed and strength of grip) were more severely impaired in patients with cerebrovascular disease involving one cerebral hemisphere or the other than in patients with lateralized neoplasms or traumatic injuries. The *consistency* of motor impairment of the upper extremity contralateral to the damaged hemisphere in individual subjects also was more pronounced in cerebrovascular disease than the other two categories. Further, a series of sensory-perceptual tests including double simultaneous tactile, auditory, and visual stimulation; tactile finger localization; fingertip number writing perception; and tactile coin recognition were included in this study. These variables tended also to be more seriously impaired on the side contralateral to the damaged hemisphere when damage was represented by cerebrovascular lesions as contrasted with neoplastic and traumatic lesions. Finally, differences between verbal and performance results on the Wechsler-Bellevue Scale, in accordance with lateralization of cerebral damage, were quite clear and pronounced in the groups with lateralized cerebrovascular lesions and intrinsic neoplasms but tended to be considerably less pronounced in patients with traumatic lesions which were judged to be restricted to a single cerebral hemisphere on the basis of neurological findings. Although these findings are presently being reported only in a preliminary manner, the results obtained suggest that there are certain rather consistent and differential behavioral deficits associated with cerebrovascular, neoplastic, and traumatic cerebral lesions. As would be expected, however, the general trend is toward similarity of deficit, with the differences occurring only in terms of relations between various types of objective testing procedures.

Our results indicate that the possibility of a degree of uniqueness in pattern, if not a distinctive pattern, of behavioral loss associated with various types of cerebral lesions would be worthy of intensive future investigation.

PRESENTATION 16

Maurice W. Van Allen

Since the presentation of Meier and the discussion by Reitan have adequately covered their assignment, I shall make my remarks brief and contribute what I can from the standpoint of a clinician.

The clinical neurologist welcomes the growth of neuropsychology. In recent decades the methods of classical examination have lost some stature as neuroradiological procedures have been developed and perfected. Classical behavioral observation has been displaced in part by diagnostic studies based on anatomical abnormalities and distortions. The accuracy of localization of many central nervous system lesions by radiologic techniques is substantially higher than that which is now reached or is likely to be reached in the near future by behavioral tests, however sophisticated.

Neuropsychology has served to revive interest in behavioral analysis. However, in the necessary concern with controls, ingenuity of testing, and mathematical analysis, those who are active in this special field should not forget that it is primarily an extension of the classical neurological examination. As such it is subject to all the satisfactions and frustrations experienced by clinical neurologists past and present. Thus, when Meier observes that "uncontrolled variables may lie outside the boundaries of immediate surveillance and control in the clinical setting," the experienced clinician can only add "amen."

These remarks are meant to add perspective and specifically to discourage the view that collaboration between neurologists and neuropsychologists is "interdisciplinary," in nature. It is not; they are at work in the same discipline.

We might consider on a purely pragmatic and contemporary basis what types of behavioral studies involving higher cortical function may be of immediate value in cerebrovascular disease (particularly since the emphasis currently is heavily on treatment) and what the clinician may reasonably hope for and expect from neuropsychology in the future.

1. The predictive value of behavioral tests is not likely to develop if one is concerned chiefly with atherosclerotic lesions. Whether value will be found in cerebrovascular disease not associated with the usual frank paralytic stroke remains to be seen. However, the clinician can expect some help now and is in need of help to clearly objectify and analyze the deficits in patients who have had "little strokes" so that the patient's residual work potential may be determined, his prognosis estimated, and treatment, if feasible, given.

Prospective studies as noted by Meier seem not to be of immediately practical value. Nevertheless, it is conceivable that a pattern of functional loss might eventually be discovered which would have predictive value and would warn of impending disaster by detection of dysfunction due to multiple small lesions.

2. The potential of psychometric tests in localization of lesions of the central nervous system has thus far not been of great pragmatic value. Nor is this a problem in which help is urgently needed in relation to the management of cerebrovascular disease, although it is occasionally of value to have data supporting the lateral localization of a lesion.

Substantial benefit to the clinician would result, however, if some help could be given in establishing patterns of deficit that would distinguish developing infarctive lesions from cerebral tumor or from primary degenerative brain disease. The progress made in this direction has been described by Reitan.

3. The establishment of patterns of loss soon after a stroke that will have predictive value in extent of recovery seems to require chiefly the application of present knowledge and skills. Such information would be of distinct value in the clinical setting and would anticipate, by some weeks, the evidence derived from less critical observation. This would be of the greatest value in planning rehabilitation programs and in supporting and encouraging the patient with significant residual skills.

4. An expansion of this point relates to differential diagnosis in regard to the nature of deficits in the stroke patient. Some recurring questions are the following: (*a*) Is he depressed or intellectually dull? (*b*) Is there a component of high-level aphasia? (*c*) Can he perform in his previous job at least in relation to technically defined intellectual functions? (*d*) Are his lesions single or multiple? (*e*) Can a postictal base line be established on which to judge improvement and future events?

In other words, help is needed to quantify and analyze the degree and nature of intellectual deficits even though important data in regard to imagination, energy, or drive may have to be derived from other sources.

In an effort to provide a simply applied tool to the patient who may be suffering from cerebrovascular disease and to quantify and objectify his progress, we are planning to study simple reaction time in patients with cerebrovascular disease. A number of investigators have demonstrated that prolongation and variability in simple reaction time are a sensitive measure of vigilance and response capability and possibly a valid index of degree of severity of brain disease (cf. Blackburn and Benton, 1955; Benton and Joynt, 1959; Costa, 1962; De Renzi and Faglioni, 1965). It is possible that this venerable tool of the psychologist may have pragmatic value in cerebrovascular disease as well as other brain afflictions.

From a clinician's standpoint, neuropsychology, at the present time, can make certain definite, important, and rather limited contributions to the management of the patient with cerebrovascular disease. There are possibilities for still greater contributions from this particular aspect of neurology. Perceptible progress is being made in the perfection and extension of the neurological examination through neuropsychological techniques and perceptible progress is being made in the understanding of brain function as these techniques are applied to lesions of nature and surgical ablations. Aided by the insights available from the other neurosciences, the advances in neuropsychology with its ingenious and well-controlled studies may be expected to provide basic information for novel and fruitful conceptions of the human nervous system. I would suggest that the next jacksonian leap in this area will be based primarily on present and future empirical neuropsychological study.

SECTION VI

Effects of Cerebrovascular Disease on Personality and Emotionality

PRESENTATION 17

Simon Horenstein

The objectives of this paper are to review the alterations in personality and emotionality which accompany or are consequent upon cerebrovascular disease and to consider the most effective methods of their management. Indications for investigative work designed to advance understanding or increase the effectiveness of clinical care will be adduced. The influence of personality, intelligence, and life situation on the clinical picture will be noted where pertinent.

ROLE OF NONANATOMICAL FACTORS IN THE CLINICAL PICTURE

Available literature provides no convincing prospective study of the effect of intelligence, life situation, and personality in a population at risk upon the timing, development, magnitude, and location of cerebral infarction (Kraepelin, 1912; Kirby, 1921; Bostroem, 1939; Rothschild, 1956; Ferraro, 1959; Chapman and Wolff, 1961; Ullman and Gruen, 1961; Weiss, Chatham, and Schaie, 1961; Wolff, 1961; Engel and Schmale, 1967; Schmale and Engel, 1967; MacRitchie and Engel, 1968). Extensive studies based on retrospective interviews confirm, as is widely believed by the laity, that such relation does exist. Data are interpreted to suggest, moreover, that postinfarctional behavior disorders are but the denouement of preexisting and determining traits (Kraepelin, 1912; Kirby, 1921; Rothschild, 1956; Ferraro, 1959). Patients whose personalities were different but whose lesions were similar, patients with similar personalities but different lesions, and healthy persons with similar personalities and life situations are not included in these selective studies. Analysis of premorbid personality is often based upon interview with family members or patients. It is likely that the premorbid personality will remain as long as any psychic structure is present, and individuals who displayed personality derangements before illness will continue to do so afterward.

Studies are needed in which prospective observations are made on a statistically valid population sample not biased by the selection of the unique. It has not yet been shown that changes in personality other than depression occur without dementia. Decompensation of prior personality traits or depression following major illness is not specific to the illness itself. Accentuation of prior personality characteristics is not unique to any form of brain disease.

Recent work raises important questions relative to the significance of personality in the generation, extent, and locus of the lesion (Engel and Schmale, 1967; Schmale and Engel, 1967; MacRitchie and Engel, 1968). Authors appropriately ask why this stroke has occurred at this time, suggesting that grave endopsychic and intrapersonal factors may influence the time at which a patient suffers a stroke. The supporting data are also derived through retrospective interview. It would be of great importance to be able to ascertain by appropriate prospective study whether one might predict impending cerebral infarction in patients at risk by the use of psychological tools. It is conceivable that combining these devices with somatic, physiological, and chemical studies might permit the development of measures leading to anticipation, modification, or delay of the infarct itself. Present information is circumstantial; yet the implications are sufficiently important to justify further study by adequately controlled experiments.

DEPRESSION

Depression of mood frequently accompanies isolated or multifocal cerebral vascular lesions as grief and resembles that observed after other major illness (Ullman and Gruen, 1961; Weiss, Chatham, and Schaie, 1961; Riklan, Levita, and Diller, 1961; Ullman, 1962). The response depends upon the patient's recognition of his loss and is accordingly proportional to his capacity to assess the magnitude and meaning of the deficit and its effect on his life. One ordinarily encounters relatively little impairment of recognition of the deficit in depressed patients, and appreciation of the significance of the alteration in body function and of the resulting changes in life situation is correspondingly high. The severity and duration of such depressive reaction appear to reflect the preexisting adaptive capacity of the patient, his self-esteem, intelligence, and experience. The environment and social milieu in which the deficit has been acquired and that to which the patient must return are also important (Ullman and Gruen, 1961; Weiss, Chatham, and Schaie, 1961; Ullman, 1962; Engel and Schmale, 1967; Schmale and Engel, 1967; MacRitchie and Engel, 1968). This is particularly well shown by patients whose loss of accustomed role and concomitant disability require them to be consigned to nursing homes. Such psychological reactions are not unique to nervous system damage or to lesions in specific cerebral locations. The reality and continuity of the loss relative to the patient's own goals play important parts. Depression thus appears quite remarkable following lateral left frontal or ventral pontine lesions among patients observed personally. The former have suffered loss of executive speech and weakness of the limbs ordinarily preferred for writing and skilled tasks, and the latter a disabling mixture of hemiplegia, ataxia, and dysarthria. Clinical accounts of their behavior note continuing depression proportional to the disability. The spectacle of such a patient grasping the lapel of the physician's coat as he mouths his speechless rage and wordlessly curses his doctor is well known. Preoccupation with self, seclusiveness, refusal to eat, striking at attendants, and crying may coincide with other manifestations of self-directed anger and loss of self-regard. Major features of psychotic depression including inability to sleep, rumination upon guilt, and attempts at suicide are usually absent. The entire reaction lightens with recovery, adaptation of the patient to his new state, and mobilization of support in the home and community. Less severely disabling lesions of the cerebrum, cerebellum, or brain stem may be followed by conspicuous though less severe depressive intervals which regress as function returns or the patient adapts. Studies in other illnesses where recovery does not occur suggest that adaptation alone may account for elevation of mood (Riklan, Weiner, and Diller, 1959). Hence, two processes, adaptation and improvement, account for recovery from depression and similar states.

The degree to which preexisting personality characteristics determine the development, intensity, and duration of depressive and allied reactions is never entirely clear (Ullman and Gruen, 1961; Weiss, Chatham, and Schaie, 1961; Ullman, 1962). Their influence appears to be reflected in the prior response of the patient to illness, injury, or bereavement. Knowledge of such reactions may help predict whether the patient will become depressed, how long depression may last, what form it will take, and how it may be managed. Depression persisting longer than 4 months appears to be unusual and is often indicative of aggravation of preexisting depression or other serious personality derangement. Persons whose previous personality was marked by obsessive-compulsive traits are particularly slow to adjust to changes in their lives. Their behavior is likely to represent a mixture of anger and disappointment. They often blame others for their illness or failure to recover and impose upon the hospital the demands they formerly made on themselves. Their hostility is rapidly communicated to medical personnel, whose angry defenses intensify the reaction. Such reactions in obsessive persons may conceal the more common grieving which may be present simultaneously.

Such environmental factors as the hospital or social setting in which the initial and extended medical and nursing care is provided, the strength of the family relations, and the degree to which plans for care after discharge coincide with the patient's intelligence, personal objectives, and ability to comprehend are important here as at any other juncture. In this sense the contribution of personal, social, and community resources to adjustment by the patient and his family appears identical to those required by any catastrophic illness which imposes continuing disability or loss. Their effective use by the physician often determines the outcome of the response by the patient and his family to the illness.

Since the occurrence and magnitude of the stroke cannot be predicted accurately, patients with cerebral vascular disease can rarely be prepared for their major losses, and hence differ from many patients about to undergo surgical procedures. Consequently, adaptation begins most often at a time when grief and anxiety are maximal and judgment most impaired.

MANAGEMENT OF DEPRESSION

The management of depression and allied conditions depends upon a program which begins after an unexpected catastrophe and considers the previous adaptive capacity, personality, life situation, and intelligence of the patient and family; the quantitative and qualitative aspects of the deficit; the meaning of the disorder to the patient and his family; and the environment in which the illness has occurred, is treated, and to which the patient will return (Rothschild, 1956; Ferraro, 1959).

The same social, psychological, and pharmacological methods useful in dealing with any depression yield comparable results when depression, grief reaction, or similar decompensation occurs after cerebral infarction. The circumstances, however, require different application of these tools. Evaluation of actual disability in the patient's personal situation is crucial to understanding the victim's response. The greater the loss of function, the more severely the defenses of the patient, his family, and the community will be taxed. Full realization of the loss often comes slowly, and the full effect of grieving or "giving up" may not be evident until relatively late, often only after the patient has passed the acute phase of his illness. The endopsychic factors which some believe influential upon the timing of the cerebral insult may also contribute to the patient's continuing incapacity to participate in the medical management and social adjustments needed to cope with the stroke (Engel and Schmale, 1967; Schmale and Engel, 1967; MacRitchie and Engel, 1968). Such patients may require direct psychiatric assistance either in group or individual therapy. In the author's experience this occurs rather infrequently, and invariably in those who have suffered preexisting personality disorders. Major character, neurotic, and psychotic disorders may be present in other patients, and in such cases the psychiatric disorder requires independent treatment when it interferes with management of the stroke.

Management of depressive, giving-up, and grief reactions in cerebral vascular disease has not been studied systematically. The steps which appear useful and form the basis of management of such problems on the neurological service at the Highland View Hospital include the following:

1. Positive therapeutic measures introduced at the onset, including the early use of passive or, preferably, active assisted range of motion exercises, a trapeze, effective and encouraging nursing, and active continuing interest by the physician, set the stage for the patient's participation in a determined and enthusiastic approach to the illness. These and like steps should be maintained into the recovery period. The patient should care for himself increasingly. This reduces dependency and its accompanying loss of self-esteem. Bathing, feeding, use of bedpan or urinal, and exercise of the affected hand and arm may be made his responsibility with corresponding preservation of personal dignity. Depersonalization from a man to a "CVA" or "left hemi" occurs easily and should be avoided. The physician must be frank and honest from the onset if he is to help the patient plan his future. Depressive and similar reactions cannot be disposed of quickly and require intensive sustained efforts at the amelioration of real factors related to the neurological deficit itself and the institution of measures directed toward the social and personal consequences of the illness. The projection of an unrealistically affirmative attitude or the offer of advice to "live with it" more often reflect the physician's reaction to his own sense of impotence than a reasonable expectation that either will help.

2. Mobilization of family and community resources should begin while the patient is in hospital. Families often exhibit reactions similar to the patient's and may require as much assistance. The same principles used in relation to the patient apply to them. Family members often want and need to help directly and may be assigned some of the nursing or physiotherapeutic duties. Investment of some of this energy often helps the family overcome its grief or guilt while simultaneously demonstrating concern and support to the patient. A major part of the emotional disorders displayed by the patients and their families appears to be influenced by the previous quality of the family structure (Ullman and Gruen, 1961; Ullman, 1962; Engel and Schmale, 1967; Schmale and Engel, 1967; MacRitchie and Engel, 1968). It is a matter of no mean concern to the patient that his family may lack the ability to respond positively to his increased dependency and be forced to place him in

a nursing home. It is of equal concern to the family that a member must thus be disposed to a hideous existence. The physician, nurse, and social worker can help alleviate grief, guilt, and anxiety by informing families of medical realities, educating them to community resources, listening to their fears and fantasies, and helping them deal with agencies, extended care facilities, and insurance companies as they make a difficult adjustment. Until patients and their families are able to make reasoned decisions, planning for the future as distinct from meeting emergency needs is pointless.

3. Functional reeducation using speech, occupational, and physical therapy should be directed initially toward independence in personal care, especially bathing and toilet hygiene. Once this is accomplished patients should be encouraged to do something for others and thus resume a more normal adult role. This may be started in the occupational therapy department while still in hospital, and once home the patient may be assigned reasonable tasks upon which others are dependent. However trivial they may be, they permit the patient to return to an adult status in which he earns a position of dignity by serving others.

4. Psychotropic drugs have, in our experience, contributed little to the recovery of the patient and are rarely required. Those which may cause postural hypotension should be avoided. Psychiatric intervention is rarely necessary.

ALTERATIONS IN EMOTIONALITY WHICH MAY BE CONFUSED WITH DEPRESSION: THE PSEUDOBULBAR STATE

Abnormal emotional expression, ostensible psychomotor retardation, reduced motility, and unwillingness to eat may create the illusion of depression when none is found upon mental examination. An apractic dementia may be present instead (Ferraro, 1959). The factors which determine such alterations of personality and emotionality appear to be anatomical and physiological. The behavioral elements may exist in various combinations. In one form, fixed facial expression, inappropriate (pseudobulbar) crying or laughing, impaired articulation and swallowing with or without spastic dysarthria or dysphagia, and degrees of mutism are attended by mood which is paradoxical to that which might be inferred from the patient's appearance (Charcot, 1877). In another, motor compulsions such as hand tapping or wringing and slowness of thought may be prominent and simulate agitated depression. Defects in learning, abstraction, and apperception may be present. Mood and mental function, though labile, are often effective within narrow, easily fatigued limits (Chapman and Wolff, 1959).

The structural lesions which lead to these states appear, *inter alia,* to affect the frontal cortex, its projections upon the upper brain stem, and its striatal connections. In nearly all documented instances the lesions are bilateral, relatively symmetrical, and widespread in both corticobulbar systems (Ferraro, 1959).

Disturbances of emotionality with pseudobulbar states do not occur spontaneously, though they may be compulsive in the sense that they are uncontrollable. There is no fixed mood, and its emotional expression may reflect neither its quality nor intensity. Invariably some emotion-tinged event has provoked joyful or nostalgic reminiscence which is followed by laughter or crying which exceeds that required by the stimulus. It may be stereotyped, as crying may be the only form of emotional expression possible, and initial laughter turns into crying. The emotional reaction appears to depend upon release of a simple and lower-level motor pattern from inhibition or modification. Patients often comment on its uncontrollable and inappropriate character. It rarely occurs in isolation and is usually accompanied by other manifestation of release of bulbar mechanisms from higher controls, such as periodic respiration, fluctuating pupils, dysarthria, and dysphagia.

Facial and ocular immobility further contribute to loss of emotional expression and apparent fixation in one (Charcot, 1877; Foley, 1968). The forehead is wrinkled in elevation, the eyelids retracted, and the smile squared as the corners of the mouth become tonically elevated. Patients may be unable to lick their lips on command though able to do so when wet, or move their eyes except in pursuit of a target or upon the evocation of oculocephalic responses. The tongue may be immobile and maintained in protrusion. The resulting fixed facial and ocular posture is often misinterpreted and assigned an incorrect symbolic significance. Such expressive improverishment acquires affective meaning only in the mind of the beholder. That of the patient may be concerned with other things.

Mutism is relatively uncommon in aphasic patients and its occurrence in the absence of aphasia or cortical dysarthria may result from bifrontal or anterior callosal lesions (Geschwind, 1964). Its severity ranges from no speech at all to grammatically correct though relatively infrequent speech of low volume. It is difficult to discern from data obtained in cases of cerebral vascular disease which lesions are crucial, but mutism as opposed to aphasia may follow surgical lesions in many locations including both medial frontal regions, the globus pallidus, and both lateral thalami (Poppen, 1939; Geschwind, 1964).

Mutism following parasagittal frontal infarction complicating attempted obliteration of an anterior communicating artery aneurysm appears to recover sequentially, and analysis of the stages may lead to understanding of some phenomena observed in hypertensive dementia.

Strong stimulation may evoke a rarely uttered though well-articulated word or phrase upon emergence from a stage of complete mutism. Later stereotyped phrases are emitted after delay, though in syntactically proper order upon direct question or persuasion. Feeble gestures and more varied and individualized expressions are next employed to indicate personal states such as hunger or discomfort. Spontaneous transactional speech recovers last, though usually partially, retaining concreteness and lacking affective quality.

Such mutism rarely occurs in isolation and ordinarily appears as part of a more general impairment of motility and thought. Maximally affected patients may lie or sit inertly for hours as visual, tactile, and auditory stimulation fail to attract gaze, alter expression, evoke prehension, or stimulate progression (Yakovlev, 1954; Denny-Brown, 1962a, 1966a). Such patients may be unable to stand owing to paralysis of the legs. Others lie for hours on end with their legs and arms dystonically flexed, though neither paralyzed nor rigid. They are usually incontinent of saliva, feces, and urine, and often heedless of stimuli applied to the body surface, responding only by withdrawal from extremely noxious or painful ones. Nutrition may become a severe problem, as they neither chew nor swallow, preferring to retain food in their mouths. Whatever "neglect" is shown is in the larger context of disordered movement.

Pari passu with return of speech, the patient begins to move his previously akinetic limbs upon contact or light pain. The movements are stereotyped, and prehension and progression rare. Postural adjustments are uncommon except upon painful or labyrinthine stimulation. Facial expression remains fixed and the eyes immobile and centered. Automatisms of grasping and sucking appear with tonic foot responses (Landau and Clare, 1966). Swallowing becomes more efficient, though it may follow prolonged chewing. Standing without help is difficult and walking often impossible as the feet cannot be freed from contact with the floor and reciprocal movement is lost. As recovery proceeds, a narrow-based gait, with progression by small paces (Brun's frontal apraxia) and paradoxical resistance to passive movement in the absence of rigidity or dystonia (*Gegenhalten*), are found (Yakovlev, 1954; Meyer and Barron, 1960). Grasping, picking, and facile distraction of gaze are now prominent. A variety of apparently forced compulsive acts including blinking, retraction of the lips and protrusion of the tongue, persistent syllabic iteration, and compulsive tapping may occupy the patient's waking hours. The apparent psychomotor retardation is now found to mask a severe disorder of abstraction with correspondingly concrete thought, emotional lability, impairment of judgment, and satisfaction with the adapted state (Wolff, 1961; Chapman and Wolff, 1961; Kiev *et al.*, 1962). The content and meaning of speech are shallow. Conversation is poorly initiated or sustained, as the patient lacks the imagination to deal with any but the most tangible. Although not aphasic in the ordinary sense, his use of language has become excessively literal. A common example is the response, "Yes," to the question, "Can you tell me your name?" The patient has failed to understand that the examiner has asked his name and concretely affirms that he can utter it. Such incapacity to recognize and use abstract qualities appears as part of the more general apractic disorder which emerges upon returning movement.

Apraxia is marked by inability to perform or conceive an imaginary or "as if" movement (Denny-Brown, 1958, 1966a; Alajouanine and Lhermitte, 1963; Hécaen, de Ajuriaguerra, and Angelergues, 1963; Luria, 1965). It is usually of mixed ideomotor form in the cases under discussion. Responses to contactual, tactile, or concurrent visual or auditory stimuli become released as responses at a distance become lost. The result is distractibility by the immediate, sedulous attention to the continuous, and simplification of serial behavior projected in space and time in response to single or widely separated, though related, events. Apraxia is thus bilateral and biphasic. Its expression may vary from inability to enact a complex performance by gesture to loss of the capacity to manipulate a utensil. Grasping, groping, compulsive palpation, rooting, sucking, and other positive automatisms may be easily demonstrated in the apractic patient upon lightly moving palmar or perioral stimulation or movement within the visual field. The hand often maintains firm contact with the bedclothing or body surface. Preoccupation with the immediate and continuous marks the mental state and appears to account for the patient's inertia and satisfaction with the condition to which he has adapted. Apractic dementia is the disorder of personality and emotionality which accompanies the pseudobulbar manifestations of extensive bifrontal lesions.

PARANOID AND DELUSIONAL DISTURBANCES; DENIAL

Systematized referential or paranoid thinking, somatic or spatial delusions or hallucinations, and autism are common consequences of focal cerebral lesions when sensory or perceptual functions are disturbed (Weinstein and Kahn, 1955; Anastasopoulous, 1963; Horenstein and Casey, 1964). Simple sensory disorders appear unlikely to be accompanied by paranoid or other delusional manifestations except in the sphere of deprivation. Perceptual disorders without sensory loss may, however, be accompanied by hallucinosis or delusion (Anastasopoulous, 1963; Horenstein and Casey, 1964). The latter's form, content, affective component, relations to a recent illness, and disappearance with recovery identify them with the disturbed neuropsychological function resulting from the stroke.

Perceptual disorders may be accompanied by abnormalities of psychological function in proportion to the severity of the neurological deficit and relatively independent of prior personality (Ullman, 1962). The common, though not necessarily only, focal lesion occupies the temporoparietal junction and its underlying white matter (Kirby, 1921; Critchley, 1953; Weinstein and Kahn, 1955). Though the infarct may be unilateral, the clinical features are bilateral (Horenstein and Casey, 1963; Denny-Brown, 1966b). In addition, the effects invariably involve tactile, visual, and auditory perception. The greater the polymodal defect, the more severe the mental disorder appears to be. Recovery parallels that of even a single modality (Horenstein, unpublished). Amorphosynthesis, or impaired "spatial summation," of the stimulus is present bilaterally, though to greater degree in the contralateral sensory field (Denny-Brown, Meyer, and Horenstein, 1952; Denny-Brown, 1963). Vision contralateral to the lesion becomes abnormal as its threshold is raised, temporal resolution protracted, and spatial localization inaccurate. The patient perceives stimuli arising from homologous parts of the visual field as "different" from one another. Amorphosynthesis of milder degree may be demonstrated in the ipsilateral field when severe on the contralateral side (Horenstein and Casey, 1963). Spatial localization, estimation of distance, opticokinetic, and optomotor responses are impaired (Horenstein, 1968).

Among the consequences of such imbalance between sensory fields is that some signals are perceived differently from similar ones arising elsewhere, and behavior acquires a bias toward one set. The outcome of perceptual rivalry between bilateral and nearly simultaneous equivalent stimuli thus becomes disproportionate direction of attention to one and imperception and neglect of the other (Denny-Brown, Meyer, and Horenstein, 1952). Extinction thus elicited is not unique to a single nervous level, as it does not require a lesion at all and may be demonstrated in normals by appropriate stimulus manipulation (von Békésy, 1967). Extinction may be compensated or its direction reversed in patients by spatial or temporal summation of the stimulus in the affected sensory field (Horenstein and Casey, 1963, 1964; Birch, Belmont, and Karp, 1964a). Extinction upon the use of nearly equivalent stimuli, the pervasive persistence of the process, and its effect on behavior are unique to cerebral disease. Release of the unaltered parts of the brain from regulation appears to account for extinction, and neglect and loss of inhibitory influences permit relative enhancement of perceived stimuli (Denny-Brown, Meyer, and Horenstein, 1952; Horenstein and Casey, 1963, 1964; Denny-Brown, 1963). Naturally occurring perceptual rivalry thus becomes biased and attention fixed upon the released field. The process usually affects multiple modalities simultaneously, involves an entire side of the body and space, requires sensation to be present in the affected field, and varies in intensity. The common vascular lesion occupies the white matter underneath the supramarginal and angular gyri. It has not been reported to persist after cortical ablation. The process may be present when lesions involve either hemisphere, though the global aphasia which follows most left cerebral lesions renders the patient asymbolic for his perceptual disorder (Denny-Brown, Meyer, and Horenstein, 1952; Denny-Brown and Banker, 1954; Denny-Brown, 1963). The outcome of perceptual rivalry is thus biased and associated with drastically altered emotional response and personality structure (Denny-Brown, Meyer, and Horenstein, 1952; Weinstein and Kahn, 1955; Ullman, 1962; Denny-Brown, 1963). The behavior which parallels the neurological deficits following a major parietotemporal lesion may be arranged in descending order of severity with the visual system taken as an example.

There is no useful contralateral vision when anosognosia and explicit verbal denial of blindness are present. Visual function is grossly defective, though residual vision may be demonstrated within the incongruously affected contralateral field. The head and eyes deviate toward the lesion. The patient, imperceptive of his loss, denies its existence and insists that his vision is normal (Bender, 1963). Contralateral amorphosynthesis is gross. Less severe ipsilateral imperception may be shown by such errors as inability to estimate distance or touch points in space (Cole, Schutta, and Warrington, 1962). Such perceptual defects rarely exist without some disturbance of tactile or auditory elements and contralateral hemiparesis. The unconcerned patient cannot account for his illness or presence in hospital. His explanations are fatuous and distorted, and he cannot be convinced of his error. He assesses distances from his body surface incorrectly, attends only to one side of space, and denies that his contralateral side exists. Objects and spatial arrays are misinterpreted, and attempts to reproduce them are distorted. He may see as complete portions of objects presented to him, read only the ipsilateral extremity of words, eat from but one side of his plate, and be unable to bisect lines or copy or construct figures (Bender and Teuber, 1946; Denny-Brown, Meyers, and Horenstein, 1952; Warrington, 1962; Kinsbourne and Warrington, 1962). Psychic function thus has changed without clear relation to prior personality, intelligence, or life situation. As such patients become more aware and less fixed on contralateral space, they may become accusatory, paranoid, deluded, or hallucinated (Weinstein and Kahn, 1955; Ullman, 1962; Horenstein and Casey, 1964). Affection of other parts of brain may be associated with visual hallucination, though functional relations are poorly defined (Messimy, 1953).

The stage of constructional apraxia emerges as awareness of and reaction to the environment return. Loss of vision is conceded, though its degree, nature, and cause are misinterpreted. The patient's description of the hospital and his reason for being there is less distorted. Neglect and denial continue, but at a reduced level. The patient now explains his difficulty by suggesting that the nurses have failed to clean his spectacles or asserts that it is up to the physician to find out what is wrong. He concedes, when queried, that he is ill, though as the result of the act or negligence of someone else. The implications of these suggestions are treated as neglectfully as the illness and hospitalization. Verbal denial, implicit in act and thought, replace the explicit denial of the anosognosic level. Since the mental content is usually accessible and often plausible, the patient's errors may be accredited by the sympathetic listener, who misunderstands the denial. Projection and displacement are the principal features of the fatuities employed to explain symptoms (Weinstein and Kahn, 1955, Ullman, 1962).

The head and eyes are directed more normally and the visual imbalance is less severe. Paralexia and constructional apraxia are pronounced (Alajouanine and Lhermitte, 1963; Hécaen, de Ajuriaguerra, and Angelergues, 1963). As a new symptom the patient may report seeing two or three objects when using either or both eyes, though only one is present. An image may persist long after presentation of an object and be projected into other parts of space. The forms of polyopia and palinopia vary considerably (Bender and Sobin, 1963). Confused spatial relations appear to depend upon the composition of the sensory field. Bright lights may appear distorted or located elsewhere, then remembered or found by touch. The patient may misinterpret a large scene so that upon looking out a window he regards the curb as too high, trees or buildings angled, or roadways wider than they were. The human face, a complex and constantly changing mixture of surfaces and shadings, loses its distinctive attributes, and the patient may fail to recognize individuals or interpret facial expression (Warrington and James, 1967). Uncertain of his own spatial orientation, incompletely aware and correspondingly neglectful of his situation, it becomes easy for such a patient to complete understanding by attributing his errors and illness to external ill-defined agents. Hallucinosis readily occurs in such settings and seems more frequent than complaints about it (Weinstein and Kahn, 1955; Ullman, 1962; Horenstein and Casey, 1964). More often it is mentioned in casual conversation or elicited by direct question. The curious dissociation between hallucinosis and concern appears to be accounted for by similar mechanisms of neglect and denial. The content of the hallucinations and delusions is highly variable and appears to reflect prior experience. A bartender who had been assaulted by a burglar prior to his illness reported to us that he had heard and seen people fighting in the hospital corridor during the night. He failed to cry out because he feared injury and referred to it casually the next day. An elderly widow reported that a bed had been placed next to hers during the night and a man allowed to sleep there. The nurses had removed him and his bed at dawn. When told that there was insufficient room for this to have happened, she contended that the nurses had rearranged the room to fool the doctors. These events were projected within the affected field of each patient. False beliefs of this sort often coincide with imperception of size, location, duration, and errors in recognizing the number of objects presented at campimetry.

Visual imbalance is less, and awareness of and attention to it more, complete when the dominant perceptual error is distortion of vertical coordinates. Anosognosia is minor and the capacity to construct improved. The patient, now able to stand, may tilt his head or body toward the lesion or complain that the world is inclined in the opposite direction. When the patient is seated, the deviation of the head is tonically maintained and cannot be corrected upon command. He cannot account for the strange appearance of space and may attribute it to his glasses or poor lighting. His writing, constructions, the angle at which he holds a book, and orientation to his bed are rotated corresponding to his displacement of the vertical (Horenstein and Casey, 1963, 1964). Delusional thinking is less prominent and thought processes and emotional reactions more relevant. He is more appropriately concerned about his continuing illness. Visually directed avoiding responses may be identified as the seated patient retracts or deviates his head from a moving stimulus.

Defective appreciation of horizontally continuous space represents a minor degree of perceptual imbalance and is compatible with nearly normal psychic function. Information arising contralateral to the lesion is treated as nearly the equivalent of that arising elsewhere. Head and eye postures are usually directed forward, and gaze is readily attracted toward the ipsilateral field on double bilateral simultaneous stimulation. The ipsilateral portion of constructions and complex fields receive more attention. Delusions and hallucinations are absent. Denial is slight, though neglect remains prominent. The patient tells without coaxing that he has had a stroke and describes his deficits, but often neglects to compensate for the described deficit. Even these levels of awareness and concern may undergo decompensation with fatigue.

Visual inattention is the least degree of disorder, and without focal significance. It is evoked by nearly equivalent double bilateral simultaneous stimulation (Bender and Furlow, 1954; Denny-Brown, Meyer, and Horenstein, 1952). It is accompanied by little behavioral or postural abnormality. Attention to both sides is nearly normal, though drawn more easily to ipsilateral space. There is relatively high awareness of the imbalance.

Somatic abnormalities may be ranked similarly. They, too, rarely occur in isolation and usually accompany and are proportional to a like visual disturbance and hemiparesis. These sensory derangements are caused in common by lesions which produce heteromodal effects. The severity of each ordinarily parallels that of the others. Neglect, denial, projection, displacement, misinterpretation, and hallucinosis mark the concomitant changes in mental function. The affected limbs and side of face and body are treated as though they did not exist at the grossest level—somatic agnosia and anosognosia (Weinstein and Kahn, 1950; Denny-Brown, Meyer, and Horenstein, 1952; Critchley, 1953; Weinstein and Kahn, 1955; Ullman, 1962; Weinstein and Cole, 1963). The patient attends exclusively to the "unaffected" or ipsilateral limbs; those contralateral do not exist and hence cannot be sick. The ipsilateral hand is both the left and the right. The paradox fails to impress him. When the affected limbs are discovered or presented to him, they are identified as parts of the body of another who has somehow been allowed to share his bed or thrust them through a fantasied window. Anosognosia, denial of limb, and autotopagnosia are reflected thus in the patient's view of himself and of the world about him. Though recognizing that he is in hospital, he cannot tell why since he is not sick. He often distorts the hospital's name and may be disoriented for time.

Less severely impaired awareness of the existence, location, state, and configuration of body parts characterizes the autotopagnosic level, in which there is impaired orientation of the body to space. The contralateral side now exists, though its location and shape differ from the other. Appreciation of pain may seem intensified in proximal portions of the limb and on the trunk. Its localization may be diffuse or even projected into space. The patient's distorted conception of his limb may be accompanied by somatic delusions (Weinstein *et al.*, 1954). He may complain that his hand has been fixed in a cramped position or that an extra finger has grown from his palm, interfering with use of the others. Localization of touch or contact is grossly abnormal. Light touch or stroking may provoke abnormal sensations over wide areas. The patient fails in attempts at dressing or grooming, neglecting to shave and clothe the affected parts. He remains unconcerned as he advances illusory explanations for his errors (Denny-Brown, Meyer, and Horenstein, 1952). The willingness to offer an explanation, however incorrect, implies some awareness of the defect, since in global agnosia there is no symptom and hence no need for explanation.

Awareness of the proximal two-thirds of the limb is ordinarily sufficient to sustain normal dressing and orientation of the body and limbs (Horenstein, 1968). Stereognosis, two-point discrimination, tactile localization, and finger recognition may remain abnormal despite adequate primary sensation and acknowledgement of the limb and the illness. Perception is then biased toward the ipsilateral hand on double simultaneous tactile stimulation. Disuse and neglect of the affected forearm and hand persist (Semmes *et al.*, 1960). Tactile avoiding reactions are prominent ipsilaterally and may be elicited from the contralateral hand as power of movement returns.

Small degrees of somatic imperception, elevated threshold for two-point discrimination, mislocalization of points of contact on the hand, and tactile inattention are the least degrees of somatic amorphosynthesis. They result in very little disorder of personality or emotional expression.

Some auditory disturbance usually accompanies the grossest forms of visual and somatic amorphosynthesis, but is rarely as severe or persistent (Denny-Brown, Meyer, and Horenstein, 1952; Denny-Brown, 1963). Improvement in general mental function often occurs *pari passu* with that of auditory perception. Few systematic studies of such auditory disorders are available, though numerous observations have been recorded briefly (Denny-Brown, Meyer, and Horenstein, 1952; Horenstein, LeZak, and Pitts, 1966). Ambient sound is referred to the ipsilateral ear without precise localization when auditory extinction is most pronounced. Double bilateral simultaneous stimulation is also referred to that ear. This transient state may be accompanied by auditory hallucinosis. Soon double bilateral simultaneous stimulation at levels comfortably above auditory threshold result in localization to the contralateral ear. This paradox is unexplained at present, but may relate to "extinction reversal" (Horenstein and Casey, 1963). Auditory extinction is best detected when stimuli are near threshold and appears to be neither a source of impaired mental function nor a major clinical phenomenon in anosognosic states. The preservation or return of auditory function appears to be an important factor in maintaining awareness of space.

There is no widely accepted explanation for projection, displacement, and referential thinking. While it has been suggested that they result from preexisting personality factors, the documentation that a specific personality type predisposes to anosognosia and the method of case selection leave one unconvinced (Weinstein and Cole, 1963). Families of personally examined patients more often regard the behavior as entirely new and are puzzled by it. That the extent of the change relates to the location, magnitude, and global character of the perceptual disorder may be inferred from the resumption of normal thought processes corresponding to the improvement in the patient's demonstrable neurological deficits. Progressive lesions display correspondingly reversed disorders of dissolution of function (Denny-Brown and Banker, 1954). Patients whose disorder more nearly involves a single modality appear to retain greater awareness and betray fewer behavioral abnormalities. Complication of the disorder by other sensory impairment, especially asymmetric deafness, may alternatively sustain mental derangement. Hence, whatever personality factors may be operant appear less important than anatomical and physiological ones.

The mechanism by which these neuropsychological processes undergo dissolution is unknown. Bilateral, though asymmetrical, perceptual changes are invariable consequences of focal lesions and appear to be determinants of the severity of the mental disorder. There is little except gross description of the anatomical derangements except in the monkey (Ettlinger and Kalsbeck, 1962; Moffett *et al.*, 1967). In particular, projections to the ipsilateral thalamus, elsewhere within the affected hemisphere, and transcallosally to homologous cortical areas have not been detailed in human subjects. A simple anatomical explanation hardly accounts for recovery. The transient and permanent physiological derangements and the mechanisms of compensation have not been identified. Study of the manner in which signals are processed and of the inhibitory or facilitatory effects which are transmitted to neighboring or remote structures may elucidate the psychophysiological problems involved (Kuroiwa, Kato, and Umezaki, 1967). Such studies should involve normal individuals, patients with defined levels of dysfunction, and appropriately designed animal models.

The relation of these disorders to fatigue, "set," arousal, and drive is unclear (Battersby, 1963). It would seem highly unlikely that limbic influences play no role; yet the way in which they determine the outcome of stimulation is undefined. Memory and learning are curiously without influence upon these patients. Though they remember what they have been told about their illnesses, they seem never to believe and rarely incorporate their knowledge into their behavior.

MANAGEMENT OF PARANOID AND DELUSIONAL DISTURBANCES AND DENIAL

The derangements described above appear in proportion to the level of the neurological deficit and pose great difficulties for nurses, physicians, family members, and the patients themselves. Since they are based upon imperception, they are invulnerable to education. Since many patients (especially those who are not aphasic) remain quite verbal and persuasive, members of their families often remain unconvinced. The consequences upon the patient, family, and environment may thus be extreme. The resulting disability exceeds that imposed by concomitant motor or sensory deficit. Environmental manipulation in which patients are placed so that familiar and predictable events occur within relatively well-preserved perceptual fields seems to be the most effective step in controlling confusion or hallucinosis. Persistent discussion with the patient is of little value, since recovery of function appears to depend upon cerebral factors. Such devices as "hemianopia" spectacles cannot be used by the visually imperceptive, as the gadgets only increase confusion, but hearing aids to correct presbyacusia or properly prescribed spectacles may enhance awareness by compensating for a peripheral defect.

DENIAL AS A DEFENSE AGAINST RECOGNIZED DISEASE

Denial of disease manifested by implicit disregard for the illness or its consequences may exist independently of any of the forms of perceptual disorder mentioned above. Its existence in the presence of explicit verbal awareness of the deficit results in a situation similar to denial of disease of any other cause or locus and appears closely related to antecedent obsessive-compulsive traits (Weinstein and Kahn, 1955; Weinstein and Cole, 1963). The unwillingness to change his life situation to conform to the limits imposed by his reduced physical capacity extends to a diseased state the patient's prior personality. Such individuals are often ones who always solved problems by denial and continue to do so after the stroke. They refuse to contemplate purchase of a wheelchair, since they are confident that they will walk again although they have been hemiparetic for months. They will not modify their living quarters since they will be able to climb stairs when they get home. In most instances this reaction succumbs to inescapable reality and may then be replaced by a somewhat paranoid depressive interval. The meaning of "denial" in this context and its difference from that attendant upon a focal cerebral lesion with imperception are readily perceived. Practical management is often better directed to the soon-to-follow depression. A few patients fail to advance and may display denial to a degree which interferes with effective adaptation to the stroke. Efforts at overcoming this by repeated interviews aimed at exploring the meaning of the stroke and its relation to the circumstances of the patient's life may succeed, but more often psychiatric assistance is required. An adjustment equivalent to that made to other losses usually follows resolution, but may require some months to complete. Denial and depression often exist in proportion to what is at stake. Patients with more to lose, especially those who are younger and were more active, appear more likely to display these reactions than older patients who have already made an adjustment to the reduced activity imposed by advancing years (Ullman, 1962).

AMNESTIC STATES AND DELIRIUM

Amnestic states or persistent agitation or delirium without aphasia, gross derangement of intellectual function or sensorium, significant paralysis or sensory loss represent another major group of behavioral disorders following cerebral infarction. Their appearance and persistence appear to depend upon extensive, often bilateral, lesions involving the medial undersurfaces of the temporal lobes (Terzian and Dalle Ore, 1955; Victor *et al.*, 1961; Horenstein, Chamberlin, and Conomy, 1967; DeJong, Itabashi, and Olson, 1968). Amnesia with little restlessness and gross disturbance of learning may dominate the mental picture (Victor *et al.*, 1961; DeJong, Itabashi, and Olson, 1968). Delirium or agitation persisting throughout the period of survival may be more prominent than memory loss (Terzian and Dalle Ore, 1955; Horenstein, Chamberlin, and Conomy, 1967). The magnitude of the behavior disorder seems proportional to the neurological deficit and that in turn to the extent of the lesion. The areas affected lie within the territory of the temporal branches of the posterior cerebral artery. Similar states may occur transiently during hemodynamic crises within the same arterial territory. Since the posterior cerebral system also supplies the visual cortex and optic radiations, unilateral or bilateral hemianopia may be present.

The effect of the disorder on mental function is grossly asymmetric when memory, serially ordered behavior, retention, and recall are impaired, and language function, calculation, and the capacity to abstract relatively preserved, though the power of concentration may be reduced (Victor *et al.*, 1961; DeJong, Itabashi, and Olson, 1968). Retrograde amnesia may be extensive and indifference, inactivity, and loss of initiative outstanding. Memory impairment may complicate other disorders affecting more lateral and posterior portions of the temporal lobe (Milner, 1967). Even though the significance of modality segregation, if any, between the two temporal lobes is undecided, there seems to be little disagreement upon the relation of the temporal lobe to memory. Lesser forms of overactivity resembling that exhibited grossly after destruction of the basal medial temporal lobe may appear with more laterally placed lesions.

Memory and other mental processes are rather well retained despite grave delirium or agitation when the hippocampus is relatively spared and the fusiform gyrus and third temporal convolutions maximally affected (Horenstein, Chamberlin, and Conomy, 1967). Startle reactions are heightened and sleep patterns reversed. The more bilateral and extensive the lesion, the more severe the effect. Uni- or bilateral hemianopia may be present. There is little denial of visual loss. The patient, however, cannot explain his noisy agitated behavior and does not regard it as abnormal. He remains relatively unconcerned about his total illness, though he may complain of his blindness. He may inhibit his agitation briefly as he answers questions, but it soon returns to interfere with conversation or examination. Language function is preserved, though visual naming cannot be tested when the patient is blind. Agitated delirium with hemianopia may occur transiently following an episode of apparent basilar or posterior cerebral artery insufficiency. When it follows catastrophic infarction, agitation usually persists until death from exhaustion.

MANAGEMENT OF DELIRIUM AND AMNESIA

There is no obviously effective or quick scheme by which these acquired disorders may be managed. Drugs have great applicability, as they provide safe and effective chemical restraint. The choice of agent must take into account the milieu in which the infarct has occurred and avoid further damage to the nervous system by provoking hypotension and hypoxia. Chlordiazepoxide and diazepam appear to be safe. Patients frequently require doses far in excess of those customarily employed and for rather long periods. Physical restraint and padding the limbs are often necessary. Hydration and nutrition require careful attention as the distractibility may interfere with eating. Manipulation of the environment offers an avenue for modifying disordered behavior as the patient recovers. Even the most careful attempts to provide a quiet, though not isolated, suitably lighted room with maximal use of residual vision fail to ameliorate the most severe delirium. Few such patients are able to return to their homes.

AGNOSTIC, APRACTIC, AMNESTIC DEMENTIA WITHOUT APHASIA, PARALYSIS, ANESTHESIA, OR AMBLYOPIA FOLLOWING ARTERIAL DISEASE OF THE BRAIN: HYPERTENSIVE DEMENTIA

Alterations of personality and emotionality resulting from one or more large focal lesions usually occur with such gross deficits as hemiplegia, diplegia, hemianesthesia, hemianopia, and aphasia. They vary with the general disorder. Global deficits in personality and emotional expression may also occur in the absence of such focal signs. The nature and cause of dementia accompanying arterial disease of the brain other than the effects of syphilis have been controversial. The issue seems to be whether any form of noninflammatory vascular disease except hypertensive vascular disease produces dementia without a gross focal sign. Cerebral vascular changes of lesser vessels in long-standing arterial hypertension are associated with multiple small lesions widely and bilaterally distributed throughout the cerebral white matter, basal ganglia, corpus callosum, cerebral cortex, midbrain, pons, and cerebellum (Eros, 1951; Ferraro, 1959; Foley, 1968). None may be so situated or large enough to produce a local sign beyond reflex asymmetry, lateralized extensor plantar response, or pseudobulbar dysphagia or dysarthria. The most careful clinicopathological correlation, moreover, fails to account for most features save those which result from affection of major projection systems. The net effect of many small lesions is, nonetheless, extensive cerebral atrophy and altered psychic function. The onset of symptoms is rarely abrupt and more often subtle and progressive. The mental and neurological disorders combine many of the agnostic, amnestic, and apractic elements listed above, though not with the intensity described for any one and with a more global effect on mental function. As a result, use of language, memory, judgment, arithmetical ability, decisiveness, abstraction, capacity to learn, visuospatial orientation, use of limbs, stability of mood, and appropriateness of emotional response become impaired, producing a new and abnormal personality. Inertia and "fixation to the adapted state" become marked (Chapman and Wolff, 1959, 1961; Wolff, 1961; Kiev *et al.*, 1962). Reflex asymmetry and abnormality, released tropisms, and derangements of gait are common (Yakovlev, 1954; Meyer and Barron, 1960; Denny-Brown, 1966a; Landau and Clare, 1966).

The clinical story is fairly characteristic. Mood lability, reduction in drive, apathy, insomnia, and impaired judgment develop slowly in a patient with hypertension of long standing (Apter and Halstead, 1951). Arteriosclerosis and diabetes may be present as well, but sustained hypertension seems to be essential (Eros, 1951; Foley, 1968). The patient may at first be regarded as anxious, irritable, or depressed. The duration of these responses to the mental changes relate to basic personality and the degree and rate of damage (Apter and Halstead, 1951). Pseudobulbar features, tremor, or other movement disorders (see earlier) may be discovered on clinical examination. Immobility of face and limbs, dystonia, fixed attitudes, flexed postures, and rest tremor may be regarded as parkinsonian, but the characteristic beating of the thumb and fingers across one another, rigidity, and akinesia are absent. Mental changes, reflex asymmetry, and released automatisms further separate the disorder from paralysis agitans.

Cerebral automatisms consisting of oral, tactile, and visual grasping and tonic foot responses become increasingly prominent as the illness advances. The gait becomes apractic. Rigidity is absent, though countermovements or *Gegenhalten* are present on passive manipulation. Compulsive movements such as lip-smacking, blinking, or protrusion and retention of the tongue occur. Tremor is usually of the action or essential variety (Ferraro, 1959).

Intellectual impairment dominates hypertensive brain disease and accounts for the major disturbances of function even though pseudobulbar, postural, and dystonic features may be prominent. There is no clear evidence why some patients display mainly pseudobulbar palsy and others dementia. Moreover, the precise determinants of the character of the personality change are unknown. Automatic behavior including compulsive touching, palpating, grasping, and regarding may dominate the resting state. Occasionally, conflicting and apparently contradictory motor mechanisms are released simultaneously. Grasping and avoiding or oral prehension and rejection may be demonstrable in the same individual though which appears at any moment depends upon prior conditions. Oral prehension is more likely to be found when the patient is hungry. Facial automatisms which include sucking, chewing, and rooting impair facial expression and articulation. Visually directed responses such as tonic fixation or deviation of gaze and rotation, flexion, or retraction of the neck distort head posture. Neck flexion may be observed in the recumbent patient, who maintains his head elevated as he gazes fixedly at the examiner. This is usually associated with palmar grasping and apractic gait. Neck retraction, an apparent manifestation of visual avoiding, accompanies other negative automatisms.

Retardation of thought and act and automatisms related to grasping characterize the clinical state when the major deficits are bifrontal. Many such patients have an awareness that they are changing and display depression. Denial, delusions, impaired effective responses, agnostic states, and automatisms related to avoiding are present when biparietal disease is most prominent. Disordered language function, exaggerated startle reflex, and hyperactivity accompany predominantly bitemporal disease. These anatomical formulations are not meant to simplify neuropsychological processes but only to imply greater disorder in one area in some cases even though there is widespread bilateral disease and global alterations of personality. The clinical disorder takes on a regional, rather lateralized bias when the arteriolar changes are more severe locally.

Though the mental changes appear chiefly to reflect the distribution of the pathology, mental content may be influenced by nonanatomical factors including intelligence, experience, previous personality, and awareness of the disease. These elements are usually obvious upon simple examination, but there is no evidence that life situation, intelligence, and personality determine either the fact or focus of dementia, nor is there evidence that knowledge of them would permit prediction or prevention of these consequence of long-standing hypertension.

MANAGEMENT OF HYPERTENSIVE DEMENTIA

Patients thus afflicted by unmodified hypertensive vascular disease present a major public and individual health problem. They constitute as much as 22 per cent of state hospital admissions and an even larger number of nursing home patients, and impose a grave though undefined emotional drain and financial burden upon their families and the community which supports them with such reluctance (Noyes and Kolb, 1968). There is no evidence once cerebral arterioles have been damaged and cerebral function compromised that any form of treatment will result in improved cerebral circulation, restoration of normal neurological function, or even arrest or retardation of the process (Hall, 1951; Heyman *et al.*, 1953; Jensen and Leiser, 1953; Vander Eecken and Adams, 1953; Wilson and Hohman, 1953; Gross and Finn, 1954; Pearce, Gubbay, and Walton, 1965; Baker, Schwartz and Rose, 1966; Rodda and Denny-Brown, 1966; Talland, Hagen, and James, 1967). Indeed, hypotension or hypoxia often provoked by medical manipulation may make the matter worse (Appenzeller and Descarries, 1964). The most productive therapeutic areas seem to be prediction and prevention.

Control of arterial hypertension has already reduced the incidence of hypertensive encephalopathy and retinopathy. These conditions are now relatively rare on general hospital medical and neurological services. The incidence of hypertensive hemorrhage appears to have been reduced, though less dramatically. Prevention, retardation, and reduction of the effects of hypertension on large and small vessels remain to be accomplished. Numerous programs directed toward early case finding and treatment already exist. The results may indicate that a course of action predicated upon early recognition and energetic long-term care offers the chief hope for reducing or retarding this illness (Masland, 1968).

Effective care of the established case is another problem. Since widespread and extensive small vessel disease and loss of surface collaterals have occurred by the time the first symptoms have appeared, it is unlikely that the state of either the cerebral arteries or the cerebral circulation and metabolism can be significantly improved. Efforts toward sustaining cerebral blood flow would seem more reasonable than those which reduce blood pressure and expose the patient to additional hypoxic risk (Appenzeller and Descarries, 1964). Steps should be taken to teach the patient to avoid hypotension, fatigue, and other situations which might result in reduced cerebral blood flow or perfusion gradients. The use of drugs and such diagnostic procedures as angiography or pneumoencephalography should be limited to clearly defined conditions. Careful attention should be directed toward support of cardiac and renal function lest accompanying disorders exert a negative influence on cerebral blood flow. It is to be expected that many patients thus managed will acquire a kind of stability which may enable them to return to family life and lead an effective and enjoyable though limited existence. This is particularly true of the patient whose illness has undergone recent and abrupt decompensation often abetted by medical meddling. Severe accompanying depression may require one or more of the psychological, pharmacological, and physical treatments available for that state.

RESEARCH PROBLEMS

The mechanisms of inertia, depression, agnosia, amnesia, and apraxia are little understood. Effective and valid anatomical studies designed to establish clear clinicopathological correlations are difficult and unsatisfactory in cases of vascular disease owing to the advanced age and unpredictable conglomeration of lesions encountered in most patients. It is always difficult to ascertain whether the new lesion alone, the new lesion superimposed upon many old ones, or toxic, metabolic, or physiological changes account for the behavioral disorder. The usual cerebral infarcts, moreover, fail to conform to the functional anatomy of the brain, since they are bound by vascular territories which cross anatomical boundaries and interrupt functionally related systems. They affect large areas of cortex, basal ganglia, and white matter with resulting disconnection within and between the hemispheres. It is for this reason that vascular lesions are so likely to disrupt neuropsychological processes. The latter are dependent upon redundant systems which are imbalanced only with difficulty. Such cases, therefore, are not wholly satisfactory for any except phenomenological study, which in turn runs the risk of becoming anecdotal. On the other hand, isolated lesions of cortex rarely produce extensive changes in personality, emotionality, or neuropsychological process. Further study of the phenomena may (1) help define clinical syndromes, (2) promote understanding of behavioral mechanisms, (3) result in improved patient care upon the application of knowledge derived from the first two, and (4) enable development of compensatory techniques. Proper study of appropriate postmortem material may unravel some of the anatomical problems and lead to experiments designed to identify physiological factors.

Extension of the description of the clinical forms of specific arterial syndromes to include their usual behavioral changes and determinants appears to be worthwhile as many of the changes described above and their significance seem unknown even to well-informed physicians and other health personnel. Such study may elucidate mental processes as well as influence management, rehabilitation, and social planning.

These patients provide our major source for the study of behavioral functions resulting from lesions of the cerebral cortex and white matter independent of anatomical commitment. The frequency with which athalamic heteromodal motor and sensory cortical areas are involved provides extensive opportunity to study the function of these regions. Modern appreciation of the significance of heteromodal as opposed to specific or isomodal sensory and motor cortex largely derives from clinical studies in such patients. Further exploration of the clinical phenomena and neuropsychological processes underlying denial and neglect may enlarge upon the interrelations among them with important applications to education, especially in areas of impaired communication. The frontal cortex is also driven by heteromodal forces, though appreciation of them is less acute than in the case of the parietotemporal junction. The frequency with which this system is also affected should permit the development of studies bearing upon mechanisms underlying apraxia, motor compulsions, and gait disorders.

As one reviews the enormous relevant literature it seems that investigation of neuropsychological phenomena has been contaminated by the bias and haste of the investigators. Those who wish to account for the changed behavior in mystical terms attribute such phenomena as anosognosia to loss of body image. Others attempt to explain behavior in terms of dynamic psychiatry with rather incomplete regard for anatomical, physiological, and psychological factors. Thus, egregious errors may be made by biased examiners who misinterpret paralectic division of the word "women" to "men" as sexual aberrations. Simple anatomical formulations fail to account for varying symptoms with common lesions, and semantic quarreling about the forms of apraxia wastes a great deal of time and energy.

The inescapable fact is that every single patient has one or more lesions in his brain. All the symptoms must represent the loss and release of function consequent upon the illness. Studies undertaken to identify phenomena or discover their psychophysiological determinants should attempt to identify that which has been lost and that released; to allow prolonged observation, freedom from hypoxia, intracranial hypertension, and the effects of drugs. Each study should permit observation for as long as a year, since our own data suggest that the phenomena are unstable during at least the first 6 months. The behavioral phenomena should always be related to the accompanying neurological deficit. In this way such study may help define the determinants of mental processes which must, after all, rest upon the structure and effective function of the brain.

PRESENTATION 18

Raymond B. Bauer

RELATIVE INFLUENCE OF ANATOMICAL AND NONANATOMICAL FACTORS IN BEHAVIORAL CHANGE

I would like to compliment Horenstein on his complete and excellent discussion of this subject. It covers management of the stroke patient well, and it covers a great deal more. It provides a complete description of the organic as well as the functional mechanisms of behavioral disorders. This overlap is understandable. It is impossible to isolate management of behavioral disorders from their cause, and it is difficult to separate the effects of anatomical and nonanatomical factors on behavior change in stroke, although it seems clear that the anatomical factors are the more influential.

The effects of nonanatomical factors such as personality, intelligence, and life situation on behavioral change in stroke are hard to isolate for several reasons:

1. Most behavioral changes related to cerebrovascular disease can be shown to be due to anatomical lesions in various areas of the brain, although behavioral changes are not always exactly predictable on the basis of the location or type of the lesion. The neurologist therefore sometimes overlooks the effects of nonanatomical factors.

2. Too frequently we first encounter the patient *after* the stroke has occurred. Thus, we have no knowledge of the patient's prestroke emotional makeup and intelligence against which to evaluate just how much change has occurred since the stroke.

3. When the neurologist sees the stroke patient on a referral basis, as is frequently the case in specialty practice, not only the prestroke but also the poststroke state may be unknown.

4. Prospective studies or psychometric evaluation *prior* to the stroke are unavailable, as pointed out by Horenstein.

5. There is a lack of definite evidence that the emotional reaction to stroke is really any different from the emotional reaction to other disabling illnesses, if only the behavioral change *not* related to organic lesions of the brain is being considered.

6. Almost all nonanatomical behavioral disorders, if not present prior to the stroke, will disappear as soon as the neurological deficit disappears.

7. It may be difficult to differentiate clearly between anatomical and nonanatomical behavioral changes, since they can be closely interrelated.

That anatomical deficits influence the patient's rehabilitation more than nonanatomical factors is shown in a study by Adams and Hurwitz (1963). They noted that about 10 per cent of all stroke victims failed to achieve satisfactory rehabilitation, and that paralysis alone did not necessarily account for this. They examined 45 "failures," in detail and listed the reasons for failure in each case. They found that 18 patients (45 per cent) presented the clinical picture of severe residual paralysis, sensory deficit, homonymous field defects with varying degrees of generalized intellectual impairment, and a correspondingly high rate of incompetence; 1 patient had occipital blindness; and 3 patients had other handicaps, such as extremity amputation or visual disturbance unrelated to the stroke. These 22 patients, therefore, were handicapped mainly by physical disabilities, with or without generalized deterioration.

The problems of the remaining 23 were different. Of these, 1 patient had poor comprehension so that spoken or written instructions conveyed nothing to him; 6 patients showed evidence of neglect of the affected limbs and another 4 disowned the hemiplegic limbs or complained of bizarre changes in them; 2 patients had severe motor apraxia; 7 had postural imbalance and were confined to a hospital owing to a combination of physical and social insecurity; and 3 patients simply refused to try to get back on their feet. Of these, 2 appeared to have infarction in the territory of the anterior cerebral artery and the third had only slight residual paresis on one side but said that at the age of 96 she was "too old to try."

Thus, in 42 of these 45 patients there was a definite anatomical or organic reason for the failure. In 3 cases the reason given was "unwilling to try." Why were they unwilling? The 96-year-old woman's plea of advanced age should probably be accepted as a rational decision. The other 2 patients, however, had severe frontal lobe damage with gross personality changes: They were described as being irritable, abusive, and uncooperative when pressed, but were affable and obliging when left alone. Thus, in only 1 of the 45 patients was failure to achieve satisfactory rehabilitation the result of nonanatomical factors.

Adams and Hurwitz (1963) listed the following 14 behavioral abnormalities which they called mental (i.e., nonanatomical) barriers to recovery:

1. Defect in comprehension
2. Neglect of the hemiparetic limbs
3. Denial of disease
4. Disturbance of body image
5. "Space blindness"
6. Apraxia
7. Motor perseveration
8. Memory loss of immediate events
9. "Mirror" and other synkinetic movements
10. Loss of confidence
11. Thorough depression
12. Too inattentive
13. "Don't want to do it"
14. Catastrophic reaction.

In my judgment, only items 3, 10, 11, and possibly 13 could be considered nonanatomical and even these could be secondary to organic changes. For example, item 3, denial of disease, exists in the presence of a definite neurological deficit which the patient can deny; remove the neurological deficit and there is nothing to deny. Item 10, loss of confidence, can result not only from a neurological deficit but from any physical deficit; remove the deficit, and the patient will regain confidence. Item 11, thorough depression, probably one of the most common barriers to recovery, may occur with any type of disability, not just stroke. Item 13, "don't want to do it," may be related to depression, to poor effort tolerance, or to old age; it is not related only to stroke.

The remaining behavioral abnormalities result from organic, anatomical, or physical defects. The alert physician should be able to recognize their source and direct treatment accordingly. Ullman (1962) in a study of behavioral changes and motivation which influence recovery from cerebrovascular accidents, comments that "the victims of strokes present a variety of unique challenges which all too often go unrecognized and therefore unheeded." The proper utilization of psychometric evaluation should help in recognizing these "unrecognized" features. It does not necessarily follow, however, that once the features are recognized, management will become that much simpler. Ullman (1961) also stated that "the needs of these patients are similar to the needs of people generally—to be active, to feel competent, and to engage in meaningful transaction with other people." He suggested that "the system of rehabilitation offered to these patients may sometimes aggravate, rather than help, the patient's own discontinuity with life about him." This is more likely if the exact nature of the patient's deficit is not adequately recognized.

I am not attempting to deny that purely emotional, or nonanatomical, problems exist or that personality traits are significant in management. Horenstein is aware of this and his report is quite inclusive. He lists as management aids passive and active motion exercise; effective and encouraging nursing; active continuing interest by the physician; promotion of self-care by the patient; preservation of the patient's personal dignity; frank and honest discussion from the onset; concrete planning for the future; mobilization of family and community resources; intelligent use of and proper timing in utilizing available agencies, extended care facilities, insurance coverage, functional reeducation, occupational and vocational rehabilitation, physical therapy, psychotropic drugs, hydration, nutrition, and manipulation of environment.

All these therapeutic aids are applicable to the anatomical as well as the nonanatomical changes. However, the physician in charge of therapy must be constantly aware of the anatomical problems. His prescription of drugs to alleviate an emotional problem must take into consideration side effects such as hypertension, hypotension, hypoxia, seizures, confusion. He must be cautious in prescribing sedatives lest the patient's condition be worsened by drug-induced confusion, delerium, or anorexia. He must realize that the presence of organic deficit may make the patient invulnerable to education, a situation which causes frustration to the patient and the patient's family, as well as the physician. He must understand that behavioral abnormalities resulting from nonanatomical factors will almost always disappear as the anatomical deficit disappears.

PREVENTION OF STROKE THROUGH MANAGEMENT OF PREDISPOSING DISEASES

What we should really strive for is the *prevention* of strokes. The following are excerpts from an editorial by Page (1968), referring to the Sixth Princeton Conference on Cerebrovascular Disease:

> There was the usual talk of mass screenings to "identify" subjects who may have, or have had, strokes, but neither the methods nor the need seemed to raise much enthusiasm, possibly because an evil cloud warns there is not much that can be done about them once identified. One wonders how many mass surveys the public will tolerate.
>
> Where do we seem to be going? My guess would be that the paramount importance of arterial hypertension and of diabetes in the genesis of stroke must shortly be fully recognized and that treatment of hypertension and hope-

TABLE 13. Diseases Associated with Occlusive Cerebrovascular Disease in 178 Patients

Disease	Patients affected (%)
Hypertension	75.8
Arteriosclerotic heart disease	51.7
Hypercholesterolemia	44.7
Hypothyroidism	38.0
Hyperuricemia	33.0
Diabetes	31.0
Postural hypotension	16.0
Anemia	13.1
Myocardial infarct	10.0
Syphilis	5.0
Polycythemia	1.5

Data compiled by John Gilroy, M.D., Department of Neurology, Wayne State University School of Medicine.

fully prevention or slowing of the rate of atherogenesis will become concurrent parts of management and prevention of cerebrovascular disease.

Too many of us still nurture the illusion that if we spend enough money, or make enough surveys, or hold enough conferences, better treatment will be forthcoming.

In line with this I would like to remind you again of the role that associated diseases play. I am not stating that all these are by themselves the *cause* of the stroke, but they seem to be predisposing factors and deserve consideration.

In 178 consecutive stroke cases at Wayne State University Center for Cerebrovascular Research (Bauer, 1967), the associated diseases listed in Table 13 were found. This information is extremely important, because, for most of the conditions listed, treatment is available. Hypertension can be recognized early and treated vigorously; hypothyroidism can be corrected; hyperuricemia and diabetes can be treated. Methodical investigation can frequently determine the cause, and proper therapy can alleviate symptoms, of postural hypotension. Anemia can be corrected. Syphilis and polycythemia can be treated.

While we are waiting for the magic formula to prevent or cure all strokes, let us at least do the best we can with the knowledge available. Let us recognize that predisposing diseases exist and that their management is important in both *prevention* of stroke and *care* of the patient following stroke. A major *educational* effort (not to be confused with research effort) could be directed toward this at the present time.

ROLE OF PSYCHOMETRIC STUDIES

In regard to the role of psychometric studies in research and patient evaluation, the following factors should be considered:

1. How much information will be gained in excess of that gained by careful neurological examination by a competent and interested neurologist?
2. If the testing is lengthy and time-consuming, how valuable is it for a screening test?
3. Will it make it unnecessary to perform some or all of the currently used diagnostic procedures, such as electroencephalography, skull X-ray, lumbar puncture, brain scanning, and arteriography?
4. How available is the psychometric evaluation, i.e., are there enough psychologists to make the test available to the average physician and patient?
5. What indication is there that the psychometric examination is reliable as regards definite localization? Is it as reliable, or more reliable, than careful neurological examination and the diagnostic procedures mentioned above?
6. How valuable are psychometric tests in predicting cerebrovascular disease or identifying stroke-prone individuals without a base-line study on each individual at an earlier age? It is difficult to evaluate a patient's subtle abnormalities in terms of anything except his own previous performance; gross defects are obvious anyway.
7. Is the psychometric test able to predict a stroke patient's ability to function on the job? Since every individual's work situation and requirements are variable, it seems doubtful that psychometric tests can give this information with a great degree of reliability.

I should like to mention briefly a type of psychometric evaluation which is being applied to the patients included in a cooperative study of extracranial occlusive vascular disease (Fields *et al.*, 1968; Hass *et al.*, 1968).

Chiefly as a result of the efforts of Drake *et al.* (1968) all patients included in this study since 1964 have been given a standard mental status examination, the Neurological Index of Mental Impairment (NIMI). This, according to the authors, is an objective measurement of some of the basic mental and perceptual processes involved in coping with the routine demands of daily living. They believe that the change, over time, in these functions provides a criterion which will enhance the evaluation of various treatment methods of cerebrovascular disease and serve as a catalogue of the natural history of stroke. They also feel that the NIMI will provide a standardized measure which will make the assessment of mental function objective and possible in a large number of patients. The test can be administered by the average physician or trained ancillary personnel in as short a period as 15 minutes. The authors state that the NIMI correlates (.80) most highly with ratings based on extensive psychological testing with regard to degree of intellectual loss and closely parallels changes in patients' status. This, combined with the simplicity and brevity of the NIMI, has resulted in the compilation of good retest data.

This test suffers from the lack of information about the patient prior to his stroke. However, the ease with which it can be administered offers the possibility of recording a mental status examination on a large number of patients (perhaps as many as 2,000) in whom the neurological and vascular investigations are also standardized and include four-vessel arteriography. In addition, a comparison between those patients who have undergone surgery and those who have not, with treatment selected in a randomized manner, will be available. Outcome information pertaining to this portion of the joint study has not yet been analyzed.

PRESENTATION 19

Clark H. Millikan

When confronted with a paper as complete and as scholarly as that produced by Horenstein, a discussant may resort to isolated comments, to a few questions including points of disagreement, or to discussion of other matters. I choose all three of these approaches.

Having presumed that the primary inquiry of this workshop concerned "behavioral changes" such as alteration in intelligence, cognition, emotional response, motivation, initiation of goal-directed action, and apathy, as well as the changes associated with neurological phenomena such as hemiplegia, aphasia, homonymous visual field defects, cranial nerve palsies, and abnormalities of sensation, I asked, during the first hour of this workshop, for a definition of "behavioral changes." The question provoked a variety of answers, and now the content of the papers and discussions presented suggests that to many participants the phrase includes every change in neurological function detectable by a professional observer. Such an all-inclusive definition is meaningless. The chairman and others might well address themselves to forming a clearer statement, for the record.

Definitions are sometimes tricky. Yesterday I became depressed for several minutes when one of the discussants said, "Some of our hemiplegic patients are being taught how to drive automobiles." In my institution, hemiplegic patients have a difficult time turning in bed and cannot even walk, let alone drive a car! I queried another, who explained, "Oh, he didn't mean hemiplegia, he meant hemiparesis."

Meier used the phrase "global neurological change," which is completely meaningless to me unless it is defined, patient by patient. Specific neurological content is of great importance: A man with a complete homonymous visual field defect on the tenth day has a 95 per cent chance of having it on the twentieth day; and if he has the defect on the twentieth day (which puts him in Meier's Group IV), he has a 99 per cent chance of having it on the three hundred sixty-fifth day. Nevertheless, the patient is likely to return to his business or professional activities. If, however, the defect is severe global aphasia on the tenth day, there may be change enough in the aphasia to place the patient in Meier's Group III or even Group II on the twentieth day. Yet, in our experience, such a patient is unlikely to return to a life of active professional or business leadership. And, of course, the greatest rate of change commonly precedes the tenth day. Definitions are important.

We have been preoccupied with straightforward clinical-morphological correlations. Where is the gross and microscopic lesion or lesions associated with a consistent clinical pattern in a frequency which suggests a cause-and-effect relation? When such a morphological change is absent, many tend to implicate a "psychological," "psychiatric," or "functional" mechanism to explain unusual or faulty happenings. Some have difficulty moving from the concrete to the abstract. For instance, some neurologists find it logical that hemiparesis, aphasia, involvement of vision, and so forth, can last for a few minutes, as a result of transient focal cerebral ischemia, but they cannot accept the notion that similar pathophysiology can produce a few minutes of memory loss, as in transient global amnesia. There is nothing new about this reluctance on the part of some to accept abnormal brain function as the background of abnormal neurological or psychological phenomena. Such disorders as chorea and parkinsonism were long considered "functional." The direction of shift in etiological classification has essentially been in one direction, i.e., from the psychiatric or "functional" to the organic.

In the term "organic," I must include what might be called the chemical-metabolic substrate of behavior. Unfortunately, there has been no time to discuss this subject and the part it may play in cerebrovascular disease. How strangely reluctant we have been to accept this possibility of a brain chemical-metabolic substrate for behavior, even though the effects of one chemical, alcohol, have been known for years. So many examples exist: the effect of hypothyroidism on intellect, the production by transient hypoglycemia of extraordinary and kaleidoscopic changes in behavior, the extrapyramidal phenomena resulting from ingestion of phenothiazines, the "experiences" associated with LSD. There has been no time to explore this emerging galaxy of facts. The next conference might well focus on such matters.

There has been no time here to discuss methods to assess the highest levels of intellectual function. A common clinical problem is to hear that John Doe, bank president, is "beginning to slip a bit." His decision-making ability is said to be faulty; something is wrong with his judgment. These bits of information come from an outside source. The results of his neurological and psychological examinations are normal. Six months later the patient returns and the changes are present for all to see. Better tests must be designed. The question of retirement or continuing employment demands attention, in the same context as the example just mentioned.

In his paper, Horenstein states that "small degrees of somatic imperception, elevated threshold for two-point discrimination, mislocalization of points of contact on the hand are the least degrees of amorphosynthesis. They result in very little disorder of personality or emotional expression." Once again there is the matter of terminology. We have observed patients of this type, actually without an elevated threshold for two-point discrimination and in some instances with subtle difficulty in right-left orientation, who appeared able to return to their occupation; yet they did not and they showed slight evidence of concern about the matter. Whether such decrease in motivation and drive is a change in behavior or personality is a matter of definition. The important point is that these patients are difficult to rehabilitate and the prognosis for their return to their occupation is guarded.

The terms "motivation" and "reduction in drive" have been mentioned only two or three times during the entire workshop, and only in passing. Have you ever had the experience of having 2 patients, with equal degrees and similar types of hemiparesis, go through a rehabilitation experience with an entirely different result? One returns to work and the other makes little progress. All assessable factors are equal. But one is making every effort; the other makes none. Can we develop methods to measure motivation? Is there a chemical-metabolic substrate for such behavior? Will we be able to influence this behavior by use of a drug? That Ritalin can change sleep patterns shows that one factor in the complex behavior characteristic called alertness can be pushed in a positive direction by chemical action.

Horenstein refers to the "denial of disease in patients who always solved problems by denial and continue to do so after the stroke." This statement coincides with the conclusions of Weinstein and Kahn and Ullman. My own experience does not agree with this point of view. Like so many excursions into premorbid personality, which attempt to establish a link to pathogenesis or to an abnormal finding, this concept remains unproved and of dubious significance. At the same time, it tends to divert attention from more fruitful lines of investigation.

Horenstein also states that "some pharmacological methods useful in dealing with any depression yield comparable results when depression occurs after stroke." Later, he says that "this has not been studied systematically" and still later that "psychotropic drugs have, in our experience, contributed little to the recovery of the patient and are rarely required." Such a variety of views concerning one subject in the same paper suggests a need for more precise inspection of the relation of depression to stroke. In this connection, I would pose the question: How many patients with cerebral infarction commit suicide? Have you ever seen such an event?

PRESENTATION 20

Richard Satran

In his comprehensive paper, Horenstein referred to Engel and MacRitchie, who have been interested in the life setting in which stroke occurs. According to folklore some people have their strokes at moments of intense stress or a sudden shock. In some of the patients studied by Engel and MacRitchie it was possible to identify a significant stress occurring minutes, days, or weeks before the patient's stroke occurred. In others, stroke occurred against a setting of chronic or long-standing and often progressive difficulties in the life of the patient. In some, no acute or chronic stress could be elicited. Depression, which has been mentioned as often present before a stroke, has been infrequently observed, although reactive depression after the onset of this illness is not uncommon. The majority of the patients studied had difficulty in expressing anger and characteristically exhibited a life pattern of hyperactivity with the need to demonstrate that they were in control of their milieu.

Physicians often fail to obtain data regarding the life setting in which a stroke occurs, though such information is sought in connection with other illnesses such as tension headaches, migraine, myocardial infarction, peptic ulcer, myasthenia gravis, and epilepsy. For the immediate as well as the future care of the patient, it is important that efforts be made to identify pertinent psychological data.

SECTION VII

Conclusions and Indications for Future Investigative Work

PRESENTATION 21

Arthur L. Benton
Robert J. Joynt

The major issues and questions associated with the problem of behavioral changes in cerebrovascular disease have been presented so explicitly by the speakers in this workshop that there is little need for a systematic recapitulation of the points which have been raised. Hence, we should like to utilize this final presentation to discuss some of the implications of the information and opinions which have been offered as well as some indications for future investigative work.

ANATOMICAL DETERMINANTS OF BEHAVIORAL CHANGE

The first question that can be raised in connection with the obvious fact that significant behavioral changes are associated with cerebrovascular disease concerns the type of anatomical alteration primarily responsible for these changes. During the course of the workshop, the view has been expressed that the primary determinant is neuronal damage or dysfunction caused by infarction or ischemia. That is to say, blood vessel lesions per se (even though they may imply some reduction in perfusion of cerebral tissue) do not lead to clearly apparent behavioral impairment. As Baker and Meier have put it, there does not seem to be a direct relation between behavioral status and changes in the vessels. On the positive side, this suggests that specific behavioral deficits may follow focal infarction or ischemia and that generalized behavioral impairment (i.e., dementia or the "organic mental syndrome") may follow multiple infarction or generalized ischemia. On the negative side, the implication is that behavioral deficit is not likely to be associated with early or less-developed cerebrovascular disease which has not produced infarction or ischemia. This second point is of considerable importance, for it suggests that one cannot expect that behavioral assessment, however subtle and sensitive, will disclose early cerebrovascular disease, susceptibility to stroke, or impending stroke. It therefore deserves close scrutiny.

Observations have been cited to show that many patients with either autopsy or arteriographic evidence of significant cerebrovascular disease did not or do not manifest functional neurological or behavioral deficits. Related observations on the preictal history of stroke patients indicate a similar absence of clinical signs despite the fact that they must have had serious vascular disease for some time before their stroke. The evidence for this state of affairs is substantial, and there is no reason why the facts cannot be accepted at face value. However, it should be noted that the reference is to conspicuous behavioral defect, i.e., defect which has clearly reduced the patient's social and economic efficiency and which is obvious to all observers. Almost by definition then, if there existed minor behavioral impairment, of which the patient was not aware or which he would be inclined to dismiss and which was not elicitable by the methods of the conventional clinical examination, it would not have been noted.

Nevertheless, experimental psychologists (e.g., Spieth, 1962, 1967; Szafran, 1963, 1965) have shown that cardiovascular efficiency and cerebrovascular status are related to behavioral efficiency on tasks involving speed of reaction, decision time in complex judgments, and short-term memory under conditions of interference. Their subjects with evidence of cardiovascular insufficiency or arteriosclerosis were significantly inferior to those with normal findings. An interesting point made by Spieth (who studied airline pilots) is that the everyday life behavior of his arteriosclerotic and hypertensive subjects appeared to be unremarkable. Nearly all of them were, as he puts it, "employed and psychologically competent in the everyday sense." Another observation by Spieth is also of significance in this regard. Studying airline pilots within the age range of 35 to 59 years, he found that the subgroup of 9 subjects with evidence of cerebrovascular disease performed at a significantly slower rate on cognitive tasks than the other subgroups. However, even this subgroup performed above the average level. That is to say, their defects were not disclosed by comparisons of their performance with general normative standards but only by specific comparisons with the performance of their peers. Moreover, as Baker and Meier have pointed out, careful studies of patients with left anterior temporal resections for relief of epilepsy disclose impairment in verbal learning and retention in these patients, many of whom are engaged in gainful employment.

Defects such as these, e.g., in speed of reaction and in verbal learning, are not grossly apparent. They are brought out by precise comparisons of a patient's present performance with his previous performance or by precise comparisons involving groups matched for age, educational status, vocational status, and other variables correlated with performance level. Their significance seems to be that they show that cerebrovascular disease which has not resulted in detectable infarction nevertheless may have behavioral consequences, albeit of relatively minor degree.

Whether this conclusion has practical clinical implications at the present time is a separate question. The opportunity to compare a patient's performance with an informative previous performance rarely presents itself. Thus, even if searching neuropsychological assessment should disclose one or another type of impairment in performance of relatively minor degree, e.g., weakness in arithmetic calculation or short-term memory, one would not be on secure ground in inferring that this is necessarily related to a recent change in status; the patient may always have shown this particular performance characteristic. The chief practical implication of the experimental findings cited may lie in their indications that the monitoring of high-risk patients (e.g., those with a history of an apparent transient ischemic episode) should include an appropriate neuropsychological test battery with emphasis on reaction time, decision time, and short-term memory for both verbal and nonverbal material.

Thus it seems that two interrelated questions should be considered as still being open: (1) does cerebrovascular disease which has not progressed to the stage of infarction produce behavioral change? and (2) if this is so, are current neuropsychological assessment procedures capable of detecting this change? The two questions call for empirical study of both a correlational and longitudinal nature (cf. Benton, 1961).

The syndrome of transient global amnesia is perhaps one in which searching neuropsychological assessment might prove to be useful. As Moossy has pointed out, its pathogenetic basis is not established. Cerebrovascular insufficiency is a likely presumption, but it has not been demonstrated, and there are clinicians who are skeptical about this and who raise the question of the role of psychodynamic or "life-situational" factors in the appearance of these dramatic episodes. As Moossy further points out, these older patients typically have associated vascular disease. With this in mind, it might be fruitful to ask whether the pattern of neuropsychological test performance of these patients would differ from that of a control group of older patients with comparable vascular disease. Specifically, the question might be posed whether their performance profile would show a particular weakness in new learning, temporal orientation, and other task performances which might be associated with the functioning of the hippocampal-mamillary neuronal complex. We can be certain that gross defects in this regard will not be shown. The question is whether minor defects, perhaps judged in relation to the level of other performances, might be brought to light.

PROBLEMS OF LOCALIZATION

Several contributors to the workshop have remarked that when cerebrovascular disease results in a small infarct, it presents the most favorable opportunity for study of localization of function in the brain which the accidents of nature can provide, since in many cases the lesions are well defined and global dysfunction resulting from edema, infiltration, and mechanical pressure is minimal. One example of this state of affairs has been offered by Segarra and Angelo in the form of the "syndrome of the mesencephalic artery." Another example is that of pure alexia without agraphia resulting from occlusion of the posterior cerebral artery, as described by Dejerine and explicated by Geschwind. The pioneer worker in this attempt to relate specific types of functional disturbance to disease of specific cerebral blood vessels seems to have been Foix (1928), who delineated the presumed features of a number of discrete neurovascular syndromes, e.g., the posterior temporal artery is the "artery of Wernicke's aphasia," infarction of the territory supplied by the posterior parietal artery leads to ideomotor apraxia.

Granted that discrete cerebral infarction does afford the best opportunity for study of functional localization in man, full exploitation of this approach requires that we be aware of its limitations and at the same time consider ways to make it maximally informative.

The employment of this correlational approach, which seeks to disclose associations between lesions of specific locus in the brain and specific behavioral alterations, requires that both the structural and behavioral sides of the equation be carefully and meaningfully described. Segarra and Angelo and Moossy have indicated what needs to be done with respect to the anatomical aspect. The behavioral aspect requires equally precise description.

There is also the consideration that a discrete infarct is not likely to appear out of the blue but occurs instead within the context of preexisting more extensive cerebrovascular disease. Regardless of whether such disease already has produced behavioral changes, the clinical picture resulting from infarction may reflect in some cases an interaction between focal and general factors. This circumstance does not preclude the establishment of specific correlations associated with lesion localization, but it does add "noise" to the system which may have to be filtered out before the correlational picture is made clear.

The circumstance just cited is a particular expression of the truism that the behavioral status of a patient with a focal lesion is determined by those parts of his brain which have been spared as well as of those which have been subject to specific injury. Another implication of this truism is that we must face the problem of variation in cerebral endowment, from both the quantitative and qualitative standpoints. This variation may be of an interindividual nature or, as Meier and Baker have shown, of a cultural nature. The sources of the variation may be constitutional or experiential. Meier has demonstrated that the Porteus Maze Test performances of American and Japanese patients differ significantly, the Japanese patients showing a higher level. This difference persists even when such determining factors as age, sex, educational level, intelligence level, side of lesion, and rated degree of neurological involvement are controlled. However, as he points out, normative observations by Porteus indicate that the Japanese population performs on a higher level than other national groups on this test. The significance of this normative fact needs to be probed, for an understanding of it may well give us insight into Meier's unusual finding.

Observations such as these bring home to us the fact that cognitive, perceptual, and psychomotor performances have cultural and experiential, as well as organic, determinants. Hence, in attempting to assess the effects of a defined lesion in the organic substrate of behavior, due attention must be paid to the influence of social and historical factors.

Given these qualifications, it is no doubt true that cerebral infarction affords the best opportunity we possess for investigating the effects of focal lesions on behavior in human subjects. Ideal or close-to-ideal cases are not always available for study but present themselves only on occasion. As Moossy has pointed out, patience and a prepared mind are necessary for the accumulation of significant information. In this context, a "prepared mind" implies, among other things, the ready availability of a battery of explicitly formulated and standardized assessment procedures which could be given to all suitable cases as they are encountered. From a technical standpoint, a significant advance would be achieved if a collation of the great variety of neuropsychological test methods which have been employed in clinical investigative work could be made available. Such a collation, in which the procedures and the results of their application are described with reference to the pertinent literature, would be of great value to prospective researchers, who could then make an appropriate selection of tests from it.

LANGUAGE DISTURBANCES AND LANGUAGE REHABILITATION

Geschwind has emphasized the great social importance of the language disturbances that ensue as a consequence of cerebrovascular disease, and he has provided us with a sketch of the aphasic syndromes associated with infarction in various areas. His outline of these aphasic syndromes follows classical lines, e.g., Broca's aphasia, Wernicke's aphasia, conduction aphasia, anomic aphasia. However, many workers in the field employ other forms of classification which, they feel, are more consonant with actual observation. Here questions of definition and of terminology arise. At the present time there is considerable divergence with respect to terminological usage among students of aphasia, and as a consequence, there is faulty communication and lack of mutual understanding. It is difficult to determine to what degree this divergence is merely a matter of nomenclature and to what degree it represents fundamental differences in opinion regarding the basic empirical facts. A determined effort to resolve this issue should be made.

Elsewhere Geschwind (1969) has outlined a number of problems in the anatomical approach to the aphasic disorders which still await solution. Certain features of familiar aphasic syndromes (e.g., the disturbance in writing in Broca's aphasia) are not readily explained by the underlying pathological anatomy. The same holds true for amnesic aphasia. Nor is it rare to find a lesion at postmortem examination which should have produced an aphasic disorder during life but did not.

The question arises whether new and more searching methods of analysis may help to solve these problems. As Spreen points out, there is a "new look" in aphasia research. Investigators have tried to approach the assessment of aphasic disorders without preconceptions and with reliable methods of measurement applied to large series of cases. In some instances, the results have confirmed the validity of some aspects of traditional classification (which at least is reassuring). In other instances, the findings have served only to perpetuate the age-old controversy regarding the unitary or multiple nature of aphasic disorders. However, in still other instances, new facts, which must be reflected in a new system of classification, have been brought to light. But the significance of the new look no doubt lies more in its promise than in its performance to date. Spreen has mentioned the possibilities offered by conventional factor analysis to discern the fundamental dimensions of aphasic disorder as well as those offered by inverse factor analysis for the disclosure of aphasic syndromes, such as those described by Geschwind. A fundamental prerequisite here is the development and acceptance of standardized assessment procedures which are valid not only within a single language community but across language communities (Benton, 1967, 1969).

However, as Shankweiler reminds us, technological improvement is not enough. There is also the problem of making the most fruitful observations from a qualitative standpoint, i.e., those that will have maximal utility for diagnosis, prognosis, and treatment.

Geschwind has also discussed the application of ancillary techniques, such as the Wada test, the dichotic listening technique of Broadbent, radioactive brain scan and evaluation of the electroencephalographic responses of specific cerebral areas to barbiturates, in determining the site of lesion in the living patient. The best of these for determining hemispheric representation of speech is no doubt the Wada test, but since this is not without its hazards, the search for other indices continues. Investigative work utilizing the dichotic listening technique has yielded intriguing results, as Geschwind and Spreen have indicated. To date, however, this technique does not begin to approach the precision of the Wada test when applied to the individual patient. Nevertheless, further elaborations of its application, of the type reported by Spreen, may augment its clinical utility as well as provide important new knowledge about hemispheric localization of behavioral functions. But this remains to be determined.

From a social and economic standpoint, aphasia is probably the most important behavioral impairment resulting from cerebrovascular disease. Yet, as Geschwind has pointed out, we lack precise knowledge of how many aphasic patients there are in the United States, the conditions under which they live, or what course the disability takes. A study designed to secure this information is surely indicated to provide the knowledge necessary for the sound formulation of any broad-scale treatment program.

Language rehabilitation would seem to occupy a prominent role in any comprehensive treatment program for the patient who has been rendered aphasic as a consequence of a stroke. Yet its effectiveness is still a matter of doubt. As the critical analyses of Darley and Shankweiler indicate, there is suggestive evidence that language rehabilitation may foster recovery from aphasia, particularly if it is initiated early and extended over a period of time. Nevertheless, it is difficult to demonstrate unequivocally a significant influence of formal language training on the course of recovery from aphasia. Nor have the relative merits of different types of rehabilitation (e.g., stimulation therapy compared with programmed instruction) been reliably assessed. It should be noted in this connection (as Diller has pointed out in his discussion of psychomotor rehabilitation) that the same lack of compelling evidence of effectiveness also applies to psychological treatment for other conditions, e.g., psychotherapy in the treatment of the neuroses and psychoses or the remedial tutoring of children with developmental dyslexia.

There are a number of reasons for this lack of clear evidence for the effectiveness of formal language rehabilitation procedures in the field of aphasia. One is the context within which these disorders appear. The aphasic patient with cerebrovascular disease is likely to be an older person and the pathological process underlying his language disorder is often progressive or repetitive. Thus, added to the slower rate of learning associated with advancing age, there is the hazard that the gains achieved in therapy may be nullified at any time by a change in the anatomical substrate. Moreover, our lack of precise knowledge of the course of untreated aphasia makes it difficult to isolate a specific therapeutic effect from what may be spontaneous recovery. There is also the consideration that, although some valuable reports have been published (e.g., Vignolo, 1965), no truly adequate study of the effects of formal language rehabilitation has yet been done. Such a study will have to provide for a fully adequate control group of patients whose language experiences are carefully monitored and whose progress is compared with that of an experimental group subjected to retraining procedures which are described in detail in operationally meaningful terms. Studies of this nature need to be undertaken. The problem is a complex one and the experimental design calls for a strict control of subject variables, procedural variables, and therapist variables. Given this complexity, Shankweiler's point that "large-scale studies to evaluate the efficacy of treatment are premature" appears to be justified. Instead it seems likely that at this time a series of intensive studies of relatively limited scope by independent teams of investigators would yield more informative results than a single broad collaborative project in which practical exigencies might well force serious compromises in respect to scientific rigor.

PSYCHOMOTOR AND VOCATIONAL REHABILITATION

The same considerations apply to psychomotor and vocational rehabilitation. In this field we enjoy the benefit of somewhat more satisfactory methods of assessment of function and "real life" efficiency than in the area of the aphasic disorders, which pose such formidable difficulties in this respect. Nevertheless, as Diller has pointed out, the course of untreated sensorimotor impairment is not accurately known, and his analysis of the present state of our knowledge shows that the same questions about the efficacy of current rehabilitation procedures exist in this field as in the case of language disorders. The need for detailed studies to answer these questions is evident.

OBJECTIVE TEST METHODS

During the past decade considerable information about the behavioral status of patients with cerebral disease has been gained as a result of the development of ingenious methods of assessment and the application of more precise conceptualization in the field of human neuropsychology. These developments have been described in detail by Meier and by Reitan, who have addressed themselves to the question of the validity of the inferences that can be drawn regarding the presence, locus, and nature of cerebral disease as well as to the possibility of short- and long-term prediction of outcome in patients seen in the early poststroke stage. The findings of Meier's pioneer study in which he attempted to predict neurological outcome from behavior assessment done shortly after the occurrence of a stroke are certainly sufficiently promising to warrant more intensive exploration of this possibility. Future studies of long- and short-term outcome, which specify both the neurological and psychological parameters in some detail, are indicated.

EMOTIONAL AND PERSONALITY DEVIATIONS

Horenstein has provided a useful analysis of the singularly difficult problems posed by the emotional disturbances and personality disorders associated with cerebrovascular disease. The fact is that the relation of nonanatomical factors (e.g., personality structure, intelligence, current life situation) to the occurrence of infarction and the resulting clinical picture is not really known, such information as we now possess being circumstantial in nature. Support for various points of view has been derived from uncontrolled retrospective studies susceptible to biased observation and conclusions. Only a critically designed research project of a prospective character can furnish trustworthy data on these important questions.

A persisting question of major importance is whether the emotional and personality deviations seen in these patients represent at least two basically different types of phenomena, namely, those disturbances which are a reflection of the patient's reaction to his realization of his disability and those which are more direct expressions of the cerebral disease process (and hence of the same order as his cognitive and perceptuomotor impairments). Effective management and treatment of these disturbances no doubt depend upon a correct evaluation in this respect. But at present we have little understanding of the mechanisms underlying dementia, depression, inertia, and denial, and informative clinicopathologic study of them is not an easy task. As Horenstein has indicated, planned future research should provide for longitudinal investigation of the patient over an extended period of time. Many of the observed phenomena of this type are quite unstable, and an adequate temporal perspective is required for adequate assessment of their significance.

CONCLUDING COMMENT

The contributors to this workshop have presented a balanced picture of our knowledge of the mechanisms underlying the behavioral changes associated with cerebrovascular disease and of our capabilities with respect to their management and treatment. Not only have questions of immediate clinical interest been dealt with, but also the more basic issues that require resolution if a rational basis for the prediction and alleviation of these deficits is to be achieved. They have identified problems which call for further investigation and have outlined research approaches which offer the promise of advancing our understanding and effectiveness. It seems clear that the primary need at the present time is to encourage investigative work of a rigorous scientific character. While this is not easy in so complex a field, it can be done.

Bibliography

Adams, G. F., and Hurwitz, L. J. (1963) Mental barriers to recovery from strokes. *Lancet 2*:533–537.

Adams, G. F., and McComb S. B. (1953) Assessment and prognosis in hemiplegia. *Lancet 2*:266–269.

Adams, G. F., McQuitty, F. M., and Flint, M. Y. (1957) *Rehabilitation of the Elderly Invalid at Home*. London, Nuffield Provincial Hospital Trust.

Adams, G. F., and Merrett, J. D. (1961) Prognosis and survival in the aftermath of hemiplegia. *Brit. Med. J. 1*:309–314.

Adams, R. D. (1959) Concerning certain psychological principles which have been derived from clinico-pathologic study. *Trans. Coll. Physicians Phila. 27*:1–11.

Adler, E., and Tal, E. (1965) Relationship between physical disability and functional capacity in hemiplegic patients. *Arch. Phys. Med. 46*:745–752.

Agranowitz, Aleen, and McKeown, Mildred R. (1964) *Aphasia Handbook for Adults and Children*. Springfield, Ill., Thomas.

Alajouanine, Th., and Lhermitte, F. (1963) "Some Problems Concerning the Agnosias, Apraxias, and Aphasia," In *Problems of Dynamic Neurology*, ed. by Halpern, L. Jerusalem, Hebrew University Hadassah Medical School, pp. 201–216.

Alexander, L. (1966) Hypnosis in primarily organic illness. *Amer. J. Clin. Hypn. 8*:250–253.

Allison, R. S. (1966) Perseveration as a sign of diffuse and focal brain damage. *Brit. Med. J. 2*:1027–1032; 1095–1101.

Allison, R. S., and Hurwitz, L. J. (1967) On perseveration in aphasics. *Brain 90*:429–448.

Allyon, T. (1963) Intensive treatment of psychotic behavior by stimulus satiation and food reinforcement. *Behav. Res. Therapy 1*:53–61.

American Heart Association (1965) *Aphasia and the Family*. New York.

AMPLATZ, K. (1966) "Angiography and Cerebrovascular Disease." Presented at Joint Conference on Cerebrovascular Disease, Honolulu, Hawaii.

AMYES, E. W., and NIELSEN, J. M. (1955) Clinicopathologic study of vascular lesions of the anterior cingulate region. *Bull. Los Angeles Neurol. Soc. 20:*112–130.

ANASTASOPOULOUS, G. K. (1963) "Cortical Functions and Abnormal Experiences," in *Problems of Dynamic Neurology,* ed. by Halpern, L. Jerusalem, Hebrew University Hadassah Medical School, pp. 423–434.

ANDERSEN, A. L. (1950) The effect of laterality localization of brain damage on Wechsler-Bellevue indices of deterioration. *J. Clin. Psychol. 6:*191–194.

ANDERSEN, A. L. (1951) The effect of laterality localization of focal brain lesions on the Wechsler-Bellevue subtests. *J. Clin. Psychol. 7:*149–153.

ANDERSEN, A. L., HANVIK, L. J., and BROWN, J. R. (1950) A statistical analysis of rehabilitation in hemiplegia. *Geriatrics 5:*214–218.

ANGELERGUES, R., AJURIAGUERRA, J. DE, and HÉCAEN H. (1957) Paralysie de la verticalité du regard d'origine vasculaire; Etude anatomo-clinique. *Rev. Neurol. (Paris) 96:*301–319.

APPENZELLER, O., and DESCARRIES, L. (1964) Circulatory reflexes in patients with cerebrovascular disease. *New Eng. J. Med. 271:*820–823.

APTER, N. S., and HALSTEAD, W. C. (1951) Psychiatric manifestations of early cerebral damage in essential hypertension. *Med. Clin. N. Amer. 35:*133–142.

ARCHIBALD, Y. M., WEPMAN, J. M., and JONES L. V. (1967a) Performance on nonverbal cognitive tests following unilateral cortical injury to the right and left hemisphere. *J. Nerv. Ment. Dis. 145:*25–36.

ARCHIBALD, Y. M., WEPMAN, J. M., and JONES, L. V. (1967b) Nonverbal cognitive performance in aphasic and nonaphasic brain-damaged patients. *Cortex 3:*275–294.

ARONSON, M., SHATIN, L., and COOK, JEANNE, C. (1956) Sociopsychotherapeutic approach to the treatment of aphasic patients. *J. Speech Hearing Dis. 21:*352–364.

ARRIGONI, G., and DE RENZI, E. (1964) Constructional apraxia and hemispheric locus of lesion. *Cortex 1:*170–197.

BACALOGLU, N. J., RAILEANU, C., and HORNET, T. (1934) A propos de la pathologie vasculaire thalamo-meséncephalique: Documents anatomocliniques concernant la pathologie de l'artère cérébrale postérieure. *Rev. Neurol. (Paris) 2:*896–900.

BAKER, R. N., SCHWARTZ, W. S., and ROSE, A. S. (1966) Transient ischemic strokes: Report of study of anticoagulant therapy. *Neurology (Minneap.) 16:*841–847.

BALOW, J., ALTER, M., and RESCH, J. A. (1966) Cerebral thromboembolism. *Neurology (Minneap.) 16:*559–564.

BARBIZET, J. (1963) Defect of memorizing of hippocampal-mammillary origin: A review. *J. Neurol. Neurosurg. Psychiat.* *26*:127–135.

BARD, G., and HIRSCHBERG, G. C. (1965) Recovery of voluntary motion in upper extremity following hemiplegia. *Arch. Phys. Med.* *46*:567–574.

BARD, P., and MOUNTCASTLE, V. B. (1948) Some forebrain mechanisms involved in expression of rage with special reference to suppression of angry behavior. *Res. Publ. Ass. Nerv. Ment. Dis.* *27*:362–404.

BARRETT, B. H. (1962) Reduction in rate of multiple tics by free operant conditioning methods. *J. Nerv. Ment. Dis.* *135*:187–195.

BARRIS, R. W., and SCHUMAN, H. R. (1953) Bilateral anterior cingulate gyrus lesions: Syndrome of the anterior cingulate gyri. *Neurology* (Minneap.) *3*:44–52.

BATTERSBY, W. S. (1963) "The Cerebral Basis of Visual Spatial Perception," in *Problems of Dynamic Neurology,* ed. by Halpern, L. Jerusalem, Hebrew University Hadassah Medical School, pp. 376–398.

BATTERSBY, W. S., KRIEGER, H. P., and BENDER, M. B. (1955) Visual and tactile discriminative learning in patients with cerebral tumors. *Amer. J. Psychol.* *68*:562–574.

BAUER, R. B. (1967) "Evaluation of the Stroke Patient with Respect to Associated Diseases," in *Stroke Rehabilitation,* ed. by Fields, W. S., Spencer, W. A., and Warren, H. G. St. Louis, W. H. Green, pp. 31–38.

BAUER, R., and BECKA, D. (1954) Intellect after cerebro-vascular accident *J. Nerv. Ment. Dis.* *120*:379–384.

BEASLEY, W. C. (1956) Instrumentation and equipment for quantitative clinical muscle testing. *Arch. Phys. Med.* *37*:604–621.

BEASLEY, W. C. (1961) Quantitative muscle testing: Principles and applications to research and clinical services. *Arch. Phys. Med.* *42*:398–425.

BELMONT, I. (1957) Psychoneurologic problems of the hemiplegic patient in rehabilitation. *New York J. Med.* *57*:1383–1387.

BELMONT, I., BIRCH, H. G., and KARP, E. (1966) Disordering of intersensory and intrasensory integration by brain damage. *J. Nerv. Ment. Dis.* *141*:410–419.

BENDER, LAURETTA (1938) *A Visual Motor Gestalt Test and Its Clinical Use.* New York, American Orthopsychiatric Association.

BENDER, M. B. (1956) Syndrome of isolated episode of confusion with amnesia. *J. Hillside Hosp.* *5*:212–215.

BENDER, M. B. (1963) "Disorders in Visual Perception," in *Problems in Dynamic Neurology,* ed. by Halpern, L. Jerusalem, Hebrew University Hadassah Medical School, pp. 319–375.

BENDER, M. B., and FURLOW, L. T. (1945) Phenomenon of visual extinction in homonymous fields and psychological principles involved. *Arch. Neurol. Psychiat.* *53*:29–33.

BENDER, M. B., and SOBIN, A. J. (1963) Polyopia and palinopia in homonymous fields of vision. *Trans. Amer. Neurol. Ass.* *88*:56–59.

BENDER, M. B., and TEUBER, H.-L. (1946) Phenomena of fluctuation, extinction, and completion in visual perception. *Arch. Neurol. Psychiat.* 55:627–658.

BENSON, D. F., and GESCHWIND, N. (1969) *The Alexias: Handbook of Clinical Neurology*. Amsterdam, North Holland Publishing Company, vol. 4.

BENSON, D. F., and PATTEN, D. (1967) The use of radioactive isotopes in the localization of aphasia-producing lesions. *Cortex* 3:258–271.

BENTON, A. L. (1961) "Psychological Projects in Cerebral Vascular Disease," in *Survey Report of the Cerebral Vascular Study Group*. Bethesda, Md., National Institute of Neurological Diseases and Blindness.

BENTON, A. L. (1962) The Visual Retention Test as a constructional praxis task. *Confin. Neurol.* 22:141–155.

BENTON, A. L. (1963) *The Revised Visual Retention Test*. New York, The Psychological Corp.

BENTON, A. L. (1967) Problems of test construction in the field of aphasia. *Cortex* 3:32–58.

BENTON, A. L. (1968a) Differential behavioral effects in frontal lobe disease. *Neuropsychologia* 6:53–60.

BENTON, A. L. (1968b) La praxie constructive tri-dimensionnelle. *Rev. Psychol. Appl. (Paris)* 18:63–80.

BENTON, A. L. (1969) Development of a multilingual aphasia battery: progress and problems. *J. Neurol. Sci.* 9:39–48.

BENTON, A. L., and BLACKBURN, H. L. (1957) Practice effects in reaction time tasks in brain-injured patients. *J. Abnorm. Soc. Psychol.* 54:109–113.

BENTON, A. L., ELITHORN, A., FOGEL, M. L., and KERR, J. (1963) A perceptual maze test sensitive to brain damage. *J. Neurol. Neurosurg. Psychiat.* 26:540–544.

BENTON, A. L., and FOGEL, M. L. (1962) Three dimensional constructional praxis: A clinical test. *Arch. Neurol. (Chicago)* 7:347–354.

BENTON, A. L., JENTSCH, R. C., and WAHLER, H. J. (1959) Simple and choice reaction times in schizophrenia. *Arch. Neurol. Psychiat.* 81:373–376.

BENTON, A. L., JENTSCH, R. C., and WAHLER, H. J. (1960) Effects of motivating instructions on reaction time in schizophrenia. *J. Nerv. Ment. Dis.* 130:26–29.

BENTON, A. L., and JOYNT, R. (1959) Reaction time in unilateral cerebral disease. *Confin. Neurol.* 19:247–256.

BENTON, A. L., SUTTON, S., KENNEDY, J. A., and BROKAW, J. R. (1962) Crossmodal retardation in reaction time of patients with cerebral disease. *J. Nerv. Ment. Dis.* 135:413–418.

BENTON, J. G., BROWN, H., and RENGLER, S. H. (1951) Objective evaluation of physical and drug therapy in rehabilitation of hemiplegic patients. *Amer. Heart J.* 42:719–730.

BEN-YISHAY, Y., DILLER, L., GERSTMAN, L. J., and GORDON, W. The Ability to Profit From Cues on a Block Design Task. *J. Abn. Psychol.* 1970 (in press)

Bergman, P. S., and Green, M. (1951) Aphasia: Effect of intravenous sodium amytal. *Neurology (Minneap.) 1:*471–475.

Beyn, E. S., and Shokhor-Trotskaya, M. D. (1966) Preventive method of speech rehabilitation in aphasia. *Cortex 2:*96–108.

Biemond, A. (1956) The conduction of pain above the level of the thalamus opticus. *Arch. Neurol. Psychiat. 75:*231–244.

Billow, B. W. (1949) Observation of the use of sodium amytal in the treatment of aphasia. *Med. Rec. (N.Y.) 162:*12–13.

Birch, H. G., and Belmont, I. (1964) Perceptual analysis and sensory integration in brain damaged persons. *J. Genet. Psychol. 105:*183–179.

Birch, H. G., Belmont, I., and Karp, E. (1964a) Excitation—inhibition balance in brain damaged patients. *J. Nerv. Ment. Dis. 139:*537–544.

Birch, H. G., Belmont, I., and Karp, E. (1964b) The prolongation of inhibition in brain damaged patients. *Cortex 1:*19–39.

Birch, H. G., Belmont, I., and Karp, E. (1967) Delayed information processing and extinction following cerebral damage. *Brain 90:*113–130.

Birch, H. G., Belmont, I., Reilly, T., and Belmont, L. (1961) Visual verticality in hemiplegia. *Arch. Neurol. (Chicago) 5:*444–453.

Birch, H. G., Proctor, Florry, Bortner, M., and Lowenthal, M. (1960a) Perception in hemiplegia. I. Judgment of vertical and horizontal by hemiplegic patients. *Arch. Phys. Med. 41:*19–27.

Birch, H. G., Proctor, Florry, Bortner, M., and Lowenthal, M. (1960b) Perception in hemiplegia. II. Judgment of the median plane. *Arch. Phys. Med. 41:*71–75.

Blackburn, H. L. (1958) Effects of motivating instructions on reaction time in cerebral disease. *J. Abnorm. Soc. Psychol. 56:*359–366.

Blackburn, H. L., and Benton, A. L. (1955) Simple and choice reaction time in cerebral disease. *Confin. Neurol. 15:*327–338.

Blackman, N. (1950) Group psychotherapy with aphasics. *J. Nerv. Ment. Dis. 111:*154–163.

Bloom, Lois M. (1962) Rationale for group treatment of aphasic patients. *J. Speech Hearing Dis. 27:*11–16.

Bobath, B. (1959) Observations on adult hemiplegia and suggestions for treatment. *Psychotherapy 45:*279–289, *46:*5114.

Bonhoeffer, K. (1914) Klinischer und anatomischer Befund zur Lehre von der Apraxie und der "motorischen Sprachbahn." *Mschr. Psychiat. Neurol. 35:* 113–128.

Boone, D. R. (1961) *An Adult Has Aphasia.* Cleveland, Cleveland Speech and Hearing Center.

Boone, D. R. (1967) A plan for rehabilitation of aphasic patients. *Arch. Phys. Med. 48:*410–414.

Borkowski, J. G., Benton, A. L., and Spreen, O. (1967) Word fluency and brain damage. *Neuropsychologia 5:*135–140.

BORTNER, M., and BIRCH, H. G. (1960) Perceptual and perceptual motor dissociation in brain-damaged patients. *J. Nerv. Ment. Dis. 130:*49–56.

BOSTROEM, A. (1939) Die Klinik der Kreislaufstörungen des Gehirns vom Standpunkt der Neurologie und Psychiatrie. *Z. Ges. Neurol. Psychiat. 167:*375–389.

BOURESTOM, N. C. (1966) "Preliminary Results of a Predictor Study in Stroke," in *Conference on Research Needs in Rehabilitation of Patients with Stroke,* ed. by Fields, W., and Spencer, W. A. Houston, Texas Rehab. Res.

BOURESTOM, N. C. (1967) Predictors of recovery from hemiplegia. *Arch. Phys. Med. 48:*415–420.

BOURESTOM, N. C., and HOWARD, M. T. (1968) Behavioral correlates of self-care recovery in hemiplegia patients. *Arch. Phys. Med. 49:*449–454.

BRADY, J. V. (1958) "The Paleocortex and Behavioral Motivation," in *Biological and Biochemical Bases of Behavior,* ed. by Harlow, H. F., and Woolsey, C. N. Madison, University of Wisconsin Press, pp. 193–235.

BRAGE, D., MOREA, R., and CAPELLO, A. R. (1961) Syndrome nécrotique tegmento-thalamique avec mutisme akinétique: Etude clinique et anatomo-pathologique. *Rev. Neurol. (Paris) 104:*126–137.

BRAIN, W. R. (1941) Visual disorientation with special reference to lesions of right cerebral hemisphere. *Brain 64:*244–272.

BROADBENT, D. E. (1954) The role of auditory localization in attention and memory span. *J. Exp. Psychol. 47:*191–196.

BROADBENT, D. E. (1957) A mechanical model for human attention and immediate memory. *Psychol. Rev. 39:*1–11.

BROMAN, T., and LINDBERGH-BROMAN, A. M. (1965) Neurological rehabilitation and long-term treatment. *Acta Neurol. Scand.* (Suppl.) *13* Part II, 415–417.

BROWN, M. E. (1960). Patient's motion ability: Evaluation methods, trends, and principles. *Rehab. Lit. 21:*46–58; 78–96.

BRUELL, J. H., and PESZCZYNSKI, M. (1958) Perception of verticality in hemiplegics in relation to rehabilitation. *Clin. Orthop. 12:*124–128.

BRUELL, J. H., PESZCZYNSKI, M., and ALBEE, G. W. (1956) Disturbance in perception of verticality in patients with hemiplegia: Preliminary report. *Arch. Phys. Med. 37:*677–680.

BRUNNSTROM, S. (1956) Associated reactions of the upper extremity in adult patients with hemiplegia: An approach to training. *Phys. Ther. Rev. 36:*225–235.

BUCHANAN, J. J. (1956) Rapid mobilization of cerebrovascular accident patients. *Arch. Phys. Med. 37:*150–151.

BUDOFF, M., and FRIEDMAN, M. (1964) "Learning potential" as an assessment approach to the adolescent mentally retarded. *J. Consult. Psychol. 5:*434–439.

BUTFIELD, EDNA, and ZANGWILL, O. L. (1946) Re-education in aphasia: A review of 70 cases. *J. Neurol. Neurosurg. Psychiat. 9:*75–79.

CAIRNS, H., OLDFIELD, R. C., PENNYBACKER, J. B., and WHITTERIDGE, D. (1941) Akinetic mutism with an epidermoid cyst of III ventricle. *Brain 64*:273–290.

CARROLL, D. (1962) The disability in hemiplegia caused by cerebrovascular disease: Serial studies of 98 cases. *J. Chronic Dis. 15*:179–188.

CARSON, R. C. (1958) Intralist similarity and verbal rote learning performance of schizophrenic and cortically damaged patients. *J. Abnorm. Soc. Psychol. 57*:99–106.

CARSON, D. H., CARSON, F. E., and TIKOFSKY, R. S. (1968) On learning characteristics of the adult aphasic. *Cortex 4*:92–112.

CARTER, A. B. (1964) *Cerebral Infarction.* New York, Macmillan.

CASTAIGNE, P., BUGE, A., CAMBIER, J., ESCOUROLLE, R., BRUNET, P., and DEGOS, J. D. (1966) Démence thalamique d'origine vasculaire par ramollissement bilatéral, limite au territoire du pedicule rétro-mamillaire. *Rev. Neurol. (Paris) 114*:89–107.

CASTAIGNE, P., BUGE, A., ESCOUROLLE, R., and MASSON, M. (1962) Ramollissement pédonculaire médian, tegmento-thalamique avec opthalmoplégie et hypersomnie: Etude anatomo-clinique. *Rev. Neurol. (Paris) 106*:357–367.

CATTELL, R. B. (1936) *A Guide to Mental Testing.* London, University of London Press.

CHANEY, R. B., and WEBSTER, J. C. (1966) Information in certain multidimensional sounds. *J. Acoust. Soc. Amer. 40*:447–455.

CHAPMAN, L. F., and WOLFF, H. G. (1959) The cerebral hemispheres and the highest integrative functions of man. *Arch. Neurol. 1*:357–424.

CHAPMAN, L. F., and WOLFF, H. G. (1961) The human brain—one organ or many? *Arch. Neurol. 5*:463–471.

CHARCOT, J. M. (1877) *Lectures on the Diseases of the Nervous System*, ed. and trans. by Sigerson, G. London, New Sydenham Society, p. 202.

CHASE, T. N., MORETTI, L., and PRENSKY, A. L. (1968) Clinical and electroencephalographic manifestations of vascular lesions of the pons. *Neurology (Minneap.) 18*:357–368.

CHOW, K. L. (1950) Effects of partial extirpation of the posterior association cortex on visually mediated behavior in monkeys. *Comp. Psychol. Monogr. 20*:187–217.

CLAYTON, E. B. (1924) *Physiotherapy in General Practice.* New York, William Wood, pp. 106–115.

COHN, R. (1951) Interaction in bilaterally simultaneous voluntary motor function. *Arch. Neurol. Psychiat. 65*:472–476.

COLE, M., SCHUTTA, H. S., and WARRINGTON, E. K. (1962) Visual disorientation in homonymous half fields. *Neurology (Minneap.) 12*:257–263.

COLONNA, A., and FAGLIONI, P. The performance of hemisphere-damaged patients on spatial intelligence tests. *Cortex 2*:293–307.

CORBIN, MARIA L. (1951) Group speech therapy for motor aphasia and dysarthria. *J. Speech Hearing Dis. 16*:21–34.

CORKIN, SUZANNE (1965) Tactually-guided maze learning in man: Effects of unilateral cortical excisions and bilateral hippocampal lesions. *Neuropsychologia 3:*339–351.

COSTA, L. D. (1962) Visual reaction time of patients with cerebral disease as a function of length and constancy of preparatory interval. *Percept. Motor Skills 14:*391–397.

COSTA, L. D., and VAUGHN, H. G., JR. (1962) Performance of patients with lateralized cerebral lesions. I. Verbal and perceptual tests. *J. Nerv. Ment. Dis. 134:*162–168.

COSTA, L. D., VAUGHN, H. G., LEVITA, E., and FARBER, N. (1963) Purdue pegboard as a predictor of the presence of and laterality of cerebral lesions. *J. Consult. Psychol. 27:*133–137.

COVALT, D. A. (1952) Rehabilitation of the patient with hemiplegia. *Ann. Intern. Med. 37:*940–943.

CRAVIOTO, H., SILBERMAN, J., and FEIGIN, I. (1960) Clinical and pathological study of akinetic mutism. *Neurology (Minneap.) 10:*10–21.

CRITCHLEY, M. (1949) Phenomenon of tactile inattention with special reference to parietal lesions. *Brain 72:*538–561.

CRITCHLEY, M. (1953) *The Parietal Lobes.* London, Arnold.

CROSS, K. D. (1967) Role of practice in perceptual motor learning. *Amer. J. Phys. Med. 46:*487–510.

CROWN, S. (1951) Psychological changes following prefrontal lobotomy: A review. *J. Ment. Sci. 97:*49–83.

DANIELS, LUCILLE, WILLIAMS, MARION, and WORTHINGHAM, CATHERINE (1956) *Muscle Testing: Techniques of Manual Examination.* Philadelphia, Saunders.

D'ASARO, M. J. (1955) "An Experimental Investigation of Effects of Sodium Amytal on Communication of Aphasic Patients." Ph.D. Dissertation, University of Southern California.

DARLEY, F. L. (1965) Lacunae and Research Approaches to Them," in *Brain Mechanisms Underlying Speech and Language,* ed. by Darley, F. L. New York, Grune, pp. 236–239.

DECKER, FRIEDA (1960) *Progressive Lessons for Language Retraining.* New York, Harper.

DEJONG, R. M., ITABASHI, H. H., and OLSON, J. R. (1968) "Pure" memory loss with hippocampal lesions: A case report. *Trans. Amer. Neurol. Ass. 93:*31–34.

DELAGI, E. F., MANHEIMER, R. H., METZ, J., BELLOS, S. P., and GREENE, F. D. (1962) Rehabilitation of the homebound in a semi-rural area. *J. Chronic Dis. 12:*568–576.

DENNY-BROWN, D. (1958) The nature of apraxia. *J. Nerv. Ment. Dis. 126:*9–32.

Denny-Brown, D. (1962a) *The Basal Ganglia and Their Relation to Disorders of Movement.* London, Oxford.

Denny-Brown, D. (1962b) The mid-brain and motor integration. *Proc. Roy. Soc. Med.* 55:527–538.

Denny-Brown, D. (1963) "The Physiological Basis of Perception and Speech," in *Problems in Dynamic Neurology,* ed. by Halpern, L. Jerusalem, Hebrew University Hadassah Medical School, pp. 30–62.

Denny-Brown, D. (1966a) *The Cerebral Control of Movement.* Liverpool, Liverpool University Press.

Denny-Brown, D. (1966b) The organismic (holistic) approach: The neurological impact of Kurt Goldstein. *Neuropsychologia 4:*293–297.

Denny-Brown, D., and Banker, B. Q. (1954) Amorphosynthesis from left parietal lesion. *Arch. Neurol. Psychiat. 71:*302–313.

Denny-Brown, D., Meyer, J. S., and Horenstein, S. (1952) The significance of perceptual rivalry resulting from parietal lesions. *Brain 75:*433–471.

De Renzi, E., and Faglioni, P. (1965) The comparative efficiency of intelligence and vigilance tests in detecting hemispheric cerebral damage. *Cortex 1:*410–433.

De Renzi, and Faglioni, P. (1967) The relationship between visuospatial impairment and constructional apraxia. *Cortex 3:*327–342.

De Renzi, E., Pieczuro, A., and Vignolo, L. A. (1966) Oral apraxia and aphasia. *Cortex 2:*50–73.

De Renzi, E., Pieczuro, A., and Vignolo, L. A. (1968) Ideational apraxia: A quantitative study. *Neuropsychologia 6:*41–52.

Diller, L., and Birch, H. G. (1964) "Psychological Evaluation of Children with Cerebral Damage," in *Brain Damage in Children,* ed. by Birch, H. G. Baltimore, Williams & Wilkins, pp. 27–43.

Diller, L., and Weinberg, J. (1968) Attention in brain-damaged people. *J. Educat. 150:*20–27.

Dinken, H. (1947) The evaluation of disability and treatment of hemiplegia. *Arch. Phys. Med. 28:*263–272.

Domrath, R. P. (1968) Constructional praxis and visual perception in school children. *J. Consult. Psychol. 32:*186–193.

Drake, W. E., Baker, M., Blumenkrantz, J., and Dahlgren, H. (1968) "The Quality and Duration of Survival in Bilateral Carotid Occlusive Disease," in *Cerebral Vascular Diseases, Sixth Conference,* ed. by Siekert, R. G., and Whisnant, J. P. New York, Grune.

Elithorn, A., Jones, D., Kerr, M., and Lee, D. (1964) The effects of the variation of two physical parameters on empirical difficulty in a perceptual maze test. *Brit. J. Psychol. 55:*31–37.

Engel, G. L., and Schmale, A. H., Jr. (1967) Psychoanalytic theory of somatic disorder: Conversion, specificity, and the disease onset situation. *J. Amer. Psychoanal. Ass. 15:*344–65.

Eros, G. (1951) Observations on cerebral arteriosclerosis. *J. Neuropath. Exp. Neurol. 10:*257–294.

Ettlinger, G., and Kalsbeck, J. E. (1962) Changes in tactile discrimination and in visual reaching after successive and simultaneous bilateral posterior parietal ablations in the monkey. *J. Neurol. Neurosurg. Psychiat. 25:*256–268.

Evans, J. H. (1966) Transient loss of memory, an organic mental syndrome. *Brain 89:*539–548.

Evans, R. B., and Marmorston, J. (1963) Psychological test signs of brain damage in cerebral thrombosis. *Psychol. Rep. 12:*915–930.

Façon, E., Steriade, M., and Wertheim, N. (1958) Hypersomnie prolongée engendrée par des lésions bilatérales du système activateur médial: Le syndrome thrombotique de la bifurcation du tronc basilaire. *Rev. Neurol. (Paris) 98:*117–133.

Fang, H. C. H., and Palmer, J. J. (1956)Vascular phenomena involving brainstem structures: A clinical and pathologic correlation study. *Neurology 6:*402–419.

Faris, A. A. (1967) Limbic system infarction. *J. Neuropath. Exp. Neurol. 26:*174.

Fay, T. (1955) The origin of human movement. *Amer. J. Psychiat. 111:*644–652.

Feffer, M. (1967) Symptom expression as a form of primitive decentering. *Psychol. Rev. 74:*16–28.

Feldman, D. J., Lee, P. R., Unterecker, J., Lloyd, K., Rusk, H. A., and Toole, A. (1962) A comparison of functionally oriented medical care and formal rehabilitation in the management of patients with hemiplegia due to cerebrovascular disease. *J. Chronic Dis. 15:*297–310.

Ferraro, A. (1959) "Psychoses with Cerebral Arteriosclerosis," in *American Handbook of Psychiatry*, ed. by Arieti, S. New York, Basic, vol. 2, pp. 1078–1108.

Ferster, C. M. (1967) Arbitrary and natural reinforcement. *Psychol. Rec. 17:*341–347.

Fields, W. S., North, R. R., Hass, W. K., Galbraith, G., Wylie, J., Ratinow, G., Burns, M. H., McDonald, M. C., and Meyer, J. S. (1968) Joint study of extracranial arterial occlusion as a cause of stroke. I. Organization of study and survey of patient population. *J. Amer. Med. Ass. 203:*955–960.

Filby, Y., and Edwards, A. E. (1963) An application of automated-teaching methods to test and teach form discrimination to aphasics. *J. Program. Instruct. 2:*25–33.

Filby, Y., Edwards, A. E., and Seacat, G. F. (1963) Word length, frequency, and similarity in the discrimination behavior of aphasics. *J. Speech Hearing Res. 6:*255–261.

Fisher, C. M. (1965) Pure sensory stroke involving face, arm and leg. *Neurology (Minneap.) 15:*76–81.

Fisher, C. M. (1967) A lacunar stroke. *Neurology (Minneap.) 17:*614–617.

Fisher, C. M. (1968) "Dementia and Cerebral Vascular Disease," in *Cerebral Vascular Diseases, Sixth Conference,* ed. by Siekert, R. G., and Whisnant, J. P. New York, Grune.

Fisher, C. M., and Adams, R. D. (1964) Transient global amnesia. *Acta. Neurol. Scand. 40* (Suppl. 9), *7:*9–83.

Fisher, C. M., and Curry, H. B. (1965) Pure motor hemiplegia of vascular origin. *Arch. Neurol. (Chicago) 13:*30–42.

Fitzhugh, K. B., Fitzhugh, L. C., and Reitan, R. M. (1961) Psychological deficits in relation to acuteness of brain dysfunction. *J. Consult. Psychol. 25:*61–66.

Fitzhugh, K. B., Fitzhugh, L. C., and Reitan, R. M. (1962) Wechsler-Bellevue comparisons in groups with "chronic" and "current" lateralized and diffuse brain lesions. *J. Consult. Psychol. 26:*306–310.

Flanagan, E. M. (1967) Methods for facilitation and inhibition of motor activity. *Amer. J. Phys. Med. 46:*1006–1012.

Fleishman, E. A. (1967) Development of a behavior taxonomy for describing human tasks. *J. Appl. Psychol. 51:*1–10.

Foix, C. (1928) "Aphasies," in *Nouveau Traité de Médecine.* Paris, Masson, vol. 13.

Foix, C., and Hillemand, P. (1925) Les artères de l'axe encéphalique jusqu'au diencéphale inclusivement. *Rev. Neurol. (Paris) 2:*705–739.

Foley, J. M. (1968) Personal communication.

Fordyce, W. E., and Jones, R. H. (1966) The efficacy of oral and pantomime instructions for hemiplegic patients. *Arch. Phys. Med. 47:*676–680.

Fordyce, W. E., Fowler, R. S., and DeLateur, B. (1968) An application of behavior modification technique to a problem of chronic pain. *Behav. Res. Ther. 6:*105–107.

Franz, S. I., Scheetz, M. E., and Wilson, A. A. (1915) The possibility of recovery of motor function in long standing hemiplegia. *J. Amer. Med. Ass. 65:*2150–2153.

Freedman, S. J. (1968) *The Neuropsychology of Spatially Oriented Behavior.* Homewood, Ill., Dorsey Press.

French, J. D. (1952) Brain lesions associated with prolonged unconsciousness. *Arch. Neurol. Psychiat. 68:*727–740.

French, J. D., and Magoun, H. W. (1952) Effects of chronic lesions in the central cephalic brainstem of monkeys. *Arch. Neurol. Psychiat. 68:*591–604.

Freund, C. S. (1888) Einige Grenzfaelle zwischen Aphasie und Seelenblindheit. *Allg. Z. Psychiat. 44:*660–662.

Fromm, E., Sawyer, J., and Rosenthal, V. (1964) Hypnotic simulation of organic brain-damage. *J. Abnorm. Soc. Psychol. 69:*482–492.

Furmanski, A. R. (1950) The phenomenon of sensory suppression. *Arch. Neurol. Psychiat. 63:*205–217.

Geschwind, N. (1962) "The Anatomy of Acquired Disorders of Reading," in *Reading Disability*, ed. by Money, J. Baltimore, Johns Hopkins Press, pp. 115–129.

Geschwind, N. (1964) Non-aphasic disorders of speech. *Int. J. Neurol.* *4:*207–215.

Geschwind, N. (1965) Disconnexion syndromes in animals and man. *Brain* 88:237–294; 585–644.

Geschwind, N. (1969) "Problems in the Anatomical Understanding of the Aphasias," in *Contributions to Clinical Neuropsychology*, ed. by Benton, A. L. Chicago, Aldine Publishing Co.

Geschwind, N., and Fusillo, M. (1966) Color-naming defects in association with alexia. *Arch. Neurol. (Chicago) 15:*137–146.

Geschwind, N., Quadfasel, F. A., and Segarra, J. M. (1968) Isolation of the speech area. *Neuropsychologia 6:*327–340.

Gibson, J. J. (1962) Observations on active touch. *Psychol. Rev. 69:*477–491.

Gilliatt, R. W., and Pratt, R. T. C. (1952) Disorders of perception and performance in a case of right-sided cerebral thrombosis. *J. Neurol. Neurosurg. Psychiat. 15:*264–271.

Godfrey, C. M., and Douglass, E. (1959) The recovery process in aphasia. *Canad. Med. Ass. J. 80:*618–624.

Goldstein, K. (1939) *The Organism.* New York, American Book Publishers.

Goodenough, Florence L. (1928) *Measurement of Intelligence by Drawing.* Yonkers, N.Y., World.

Goodglass, H., and Berko, J. (1960) Agrammatism and inflectional morphology in English. *J. Speech Hearing Res. 3:*257–267.

Goodglass, H., and Hunt, J. (1953) Grammatical complexity and aphasic speech. *Word, 14:*197–207.

Goodkin, R. (1966) Case studies in behavioral research in rehabilitation. *Percept. Motor Skills 23:*171–182.

Gordon, E. E., and Kohn, K. H. (1966) Evaluation of rehabilitation methods in the hemiplegic patient. *J. Chronic Dis. 19:*3–16.

Gordon, E. E., Kohn, K., Sloan, J., Gimble, A., Grunes, J., Robinson, R. A., Mendkoff, E., Peavyhouse, B., Anderson, J., Wagner, D., Roberts, L., Young, R., and Elfenbaum, H. (1962) A study of rehabilitation potential in nursing home patients over 65 years. *J. Chronic Dis. 15:*311–326.

Gowers, W. R. (1888) *A Manual of Diseases of the Nervous System.* London, Churchill.

Grassi, J. R. (1953) *The Grassi Block Substitution Test for Measuring Organic Brain Pathology.* Springfield, Ill., Thomas.

Greenberg, F. R. (1963) "An Investigation of Paired-Associates Learning in Adult Dysphasic Subjects." Ph.D. Dissertation, University of Iowa.

Gross, M., and Finn, M. H. P. (1954) Oral Metrazol therapy in psychotic senile and arteriosclerotic patients. *J. Amer. Geriat. Soc. 2:*514–518.

Gruen, A. (1962) Psychologic aging as a pre-existing factor in strokes. *J. Nerv. Ment. Dis. 134:*109–116.

Gruenewald, D., and Fromm, E. (1967) Hypnosis, simulation, and brain-damage. *J. Abnorm. Soc. Psychol. 72:*191–192.

Guertin, W. H., and Jenkins, R. L. (1956) A transposed factor analysis of a group of schizophrenic patients. *J. Clin. Psychol. 12:*64–68.

Gurdjian, E. S., Lindner, D. M., Hardy, W. G., and Webster, J. E. (1960) Cerebrovascular disease: An analysis of 600 cases. *Neurology (Minneap.) 10:*372–380.

Hague, Harriet R. (1959) An investigation of abstract behavior in patients with cerebrovascular accidents. *Amer. J. Occup. Therapy 13:*83–87.

Hall, M. N. (1951) Study on effect of Priscoline on patients with psychosis due to cerebral arteriosclerosis. *Conn. M. J. 15:*385–389.

Halstead, W. C. (1947) *Brain and Intelligence: A Quantitative Study of the Frontal Lobes.* Chicago, University of Chicago Press.

Harcum, E. R. (1967) The parallel functions of serial learning and tachistoscopic pattern perception. *Psychol. Rev. 74:*51–62.

Harris, R., Bruk, M. I., and Copp, E. P. (1964) Rehabilitation and resettlement in hemiplegia. *Ann. Phys. Med. 7:*209–224.

Harris, T. H., and Towler, M. L. (1955) "Intracerebral Vascular Disease," in *Clinical Neurology,* ed. by Baker, A. B. New York, Hoeber, vol. 1, pp. 470–536.

Hass, W. K., Fields, W. S., North, R. R., Krichef, I. I., Chase, N. E., and Bauer, R. B. (1968) Joint study of extracranial arterial occlusion. II. Arteriography techniques, sites and complications. *J. Amer. Med. Ass. 203:*961–968.

Hastings, A. E. (1965) Patterns of motor function in adult hemiplegia. *Arch. Phys. Med. 46:*255–261.

Hathaway, S. R., and McKinley, J. C. (1951) *The Minnesota Multiphasic Personality Inventory, Revised Manual.* New York, The Psychological Corporation.

Hausmanowa-Petrusewicz, I. (1959) Interaction in simultaneous motor functions. *Arch. Neurol. Psychiat. 81:*173–181.

Hécaen, H. (1962) "Clinical Symptomatology in Right and Left Hemisphere Lesions," in *Interhemispheric Relations and Cerebral Dominance,* ed. by Mountcastle, V. B. Baltimore, Johns Hopkins Press.

Hécaen, H., de Ajuriaguerra, J., and Angelergues, R. (1963) "Apraxia and Its Various Aspects," in *Problems of Dynamic Neurology,* ed. by Halpern, L. Jerusalem, Hadassah Hebrew University Medical School, pp. 217–230.

Heilbrun, A. B. (1956) Psychological test performance as a function of lateral localization of cerebral lesion. *J. Comp. Physiol. Psychol. 49:*10–14.

Hernández-Peon, R. (1964) Psychiatric implications of neurophysiologic research. *Bull. Menninger Clin. 28:*165–185.

HERON, W. (1957) Perception as a function of retinal locus and attention. *Amer. J. Psychol. 70*:38–48.

HEYMAN, A., PATTERSON, J. L. JR., DUKE, T. W., and BATTEY, L. L. (1953) Cerebral circulation and metabolism in arteriosclerotic and hypertensive cerebrovascular disease: With observations on effects of inhalation of different concentrations of oxygen. *New Eng. J. Med. 249*:223–229.

HILGARD, E. R., and BOWER, G. (1966) *Theories of Learning*, 3rd ed. New York, Appleton.

HIRT, S. (1967) Historical bases for therapeutic exercise. *Amer. J. Phys. Med.* 32–40.

HOBERMAN, M., and SPRINGER, C. F. (1958) Rehabilitation of the "permanently and totally disabled" patient. *Arch. Phys. Med. 39*:235–240.

HORENSTEIN, S. (1968) The bilateral abnormality of opticokinetic nystagmus. *Trans. Amer. Neurol. Ass. 93*:222–224.

HORENSTEIN, S., and CASEY, T. R. (1963) Perceptual defects in both visual fields in attention hemianopia. *Trans. Amer. Neurol. Ass. 88*:60–64.

HORENSTEIN, S., and CASEY, T. R. (1964) Paropsis associated with hemianopia. *Trans. Amer. Neurol. Ass. 89*:204–206.

HORENSTEIN, S., CHAMBERLIN, W., and CONOMY, J. (1967) Infarction of the fusiform and calcarine regions: Agitated delirium and hemianopia. *Trans. Amer. Neurol. Ass. 92*:85–89.

HORENSTEIN, S., LE ZAK, R., and PITTS, W. (1966) Temporal tone discrimination in auditory agnosia. *Trans. Amer. Neurol. Ass. 91*:251–253.

HOUCHIN, T. D., and DELANO, PHYLLIS J. (1964) *How To Help Adults with Aphasia.* Washington, D.C., Public Affairs Press.

HOVEY, B. I. (1961) An analysis of figure rotations. *J. Consult. Psychol. 25*:21–25.

HOWARD, J. A. (1960) "A Demonstration and Research Study of the Rehabilitation of the Physically Rehabilitated Hemiplegic in a Workshop Setting." Report to the U.S. Office of Vocational Rehabilitation, Washington, D.C.

HOWES, D. H. (1964) "Application of the Word-Frequency Concept to Aphasia," in *Disorders of Language*, ed. by De Reuck, A. V. S., and O'Connor, M. Boston, Little, pp. 47–75.

HOWES, D., and GESCHWIND, N. (1964) "Quantitative Studies of Aphasic Language," in *Disorders of Communication*, ed. by Rioch, D. M., and Weinstein, E. A. Association for Research in Nervous and Mental Diseases Monographs. *42*:229–244.

HUNT, J. MCV., and COFER, C. (1944) "Psychological Deficit," in *Personality and the Behavior Disorders*, ed. by Hunt, J. McV. New York, Ronald Press, pp. 971–1032.

HUSE, M. M., and PARSONS, O. A. (1965) Pursuit-rotor performance in the brain-damaged. *J. Abnorm. Psychol. 70*:350–359.

JACKSON, J. H. (1879) On affections of speech from disease of the brain. *Brain 2:*323–356.

JACKSON, J. H. (1894) The factors of insanities. *Med. Press Circular 2:*615. Reprinted in *Selected Writings of John Hughlings Jackson.* London, Hodder and Stoughton, vol. 2, pp. 411–421.

JELLINGER, K., GERSTENBRAND, F., and PATEISKY, K. (1963) Die protrahierete Form der posttraumatischen Encephalopathie. *Nervenarzt 34:*145–159.

JENSEN, E. H., and LEISER, R. (1953) Use of oral Metrazol in psychosis with cerebral arteriosclerosis. *J. Mich. Med. Soc. 52:*734–736.

JOHNSON, F. H. (1953) Neuro-anatomical tracts considered as correlates of the ascending reticular activating system in the cat. *Anat. Rec. 115:*327–328.

JONES, L. V., and WEPMAN, J. M. (1961) Dimensions of language performance in aphasia. *J. Speech Hearing Res. 4:*222–232.

JOYNT, R. J., and BENTON, A. L. (1964) The memoir of Marc Dax on aphasia. *Neurology (Minneap.) 14:*851–854.

KABAT, H. (1961) "Proprioceptive Facilitation in Therapeutic Exercise," in *Therapeutic Exercise,* ed. by Licht, S. New Haven, Elizabeth Licht, Ch. 13.

KAPLAN, H. A., and FORD, D. H. (1966) *The Brain Vascular System.* Amsterdam, Elsevier.

KEITH, R. L., and DARLEY, F. L. (1967) The use of a specific electric board in rehabilitation of the aphasic patient. *J. Speech Hearing Dis. 32:*148–53.

KELMAN, H. R., and MULLER, J. N. (1962) Rehabilitation of nursing home residents. *Geriatrics 17:*402–411.

KELMAN, H. R., and WILLNER, A. (1962) Problems in measurement and evaluation of rehabilitation. *Arch. Phys. Med. 43:*172–180.

KEMPER, T. L., and ROMANUL, F. C. (1967) State resembling akinetic mutism in basilar artery occlusion. *Neurology (Minneap.) 17:*74–80.

KEMPINSKY, W. H. (1966) Vascular and neuronal factors in diaschisis with focal cerebral ischemia. *Ass. Res. Nerv. Ment. Dis. 41:*92–115.

KENDRICK, J. F., and GIBBS, F. A. (1958) Interrelations of mesial temporal and orbital frontal areas revealed by strychnine spikes. *Arch. Neurol. Psychiat. 79:*518–524.

KENNARD, M. A. (1939) Alterations in response to visual stimuli following lesions of frontal lobe in monkeys. *Arch. Neurol. Psychiat. 41:*1153–1165.

KIEFFER, S., and TAKEYA, Y. (1968) "Comparative Investigation of Angiographic Findings Associated with Cerebrovascular Disease in the United States and Japan." Joint Conference on Cerebrovascular Disease, Honolulu, Hawaii.

KIEV, A., CHAPMAN, L. F., GUTHRIE, T. C. and WOLFF, H. G. (1962) Highest integrative functions and diffuse cerebral atrophy. *Neurology (Minneap.) 12:*385–393.

KIMURA, DOREEN (1961) Cerebral dominance and the perception of verbal stimuli. *Canad. J. Psychol. 15:*166–171.

Kimura, Doreen (1963) Right temporal-lobe damage. *Arch. Neurol. 8:*264–271.

Kimura, Doreen (1964) Left-right differences in the perception of melodies. *Quart. J. Exp. Psychol. 14:*355–358.

Kimura, Doreen (1967) Functional asymmetry of the brain in dichotic listening. *Cortex 3:*163–178.

Kinsbourne, M., and Warrington, E. K. (1962) A variety of reading disability associated with right hemisphere lesions. *J. Neurol. Neurosurg. Psychiat. 25:*339–344.

Kirby, G. H. (1921) Some problems of the mental reaction types associated with organic brain diseases. *State Hosp. Quart. (New York) 6:*467–480.

Kirkner, F. J., Dorcus, R. M., and Seacat, Gloria (1953) Hypnotic motivation of vocalization in an organic motor aphasia case. *J. Clin. Exp. Hypnosis 1:*47–49.

Klebanoff, S. G., Singer, J. L., and Wilensky, H. (1954) Psychological consequences of brain lesions and ablations. *Psychol. Bull. 51:*1–41.

Klee, A. (1961) Akinetic mutism: Review of literature and report of a case. *J. Nerv. Ment. Dis. 133:*536–553.

Klüver, H., and Bucy, P. C. (1938) An analysis of certain effects of bilateral temporal lobectomy in the rhesus monkey, with special reference to "psychic blindness." *J. Psychol. 5:*33–54.

Knapp, M. E. (1959) Problems in rehabilitation of the hemiplegic patient. *J. Amer. Med. Ass. 169:*224–229.

Kouindjy, P. (1920) Reeducation of hemiplegics and their psychotherapeutic treatment. *New York Med. J. 111:*884–887.

Kraepelin, E. (1912) *Textbook of Psychiatry,* 8th ed. Leipzig, Barth.

Kuroiwa, Y., Kato, M., and Umezaki, H. (1967) "Computer Analysis of Cortical-Evoked Potentials—Application to Agnostic Syndrome Study." In *Proceedings, Second Asian and Oceanian Congress of Neurology,* Melbourne, Australia.

Landau, W. M., and Clare, M. H. (1966) Pathophysiology of the tonic innervation phenomenon in the foot. *Arch. Neurol. (Chicago) 15:*252–263.

Lawson, I. R. (1962) Visual-spatial neglect in lesions of the right cerebral hemisphere: A study of recovery. *Neurology (Minneap.) 12:*23–33.

Lawson, J. S., McGhie, A., and Chapman, J. (1967) Distractibility in schizophrenia and organic cerebral disease. *Brit. J. Psychiat. 113:*527–535.

Lazorthes, G. (1961) *Vascularisation et Circulation Cérébrales.* Paris, Masson.

Lechi, A., and Macchi, G. (1967) Mid-diencephalic necrosis during a subacute meningoencephalitis: Clinical and autoptic findings. *Acta Neurol. Belg. 67:*475–490.

LEE, P. R., GROCH, S., UNTEREKER, J., SILSON, J., DASCO, M. M., FELDMAN, D. J., MONAHAN, K., and RUSK, H. A. (1958) "An Evaluation of Rehabilitation of Patients with Hemiparesis or Hemiplegia Due to Cerebrovascular Disease," in Rehabilitation Monograph XV. New York, Institute of Physical Medicine and Rehabilitation, New York Univ.

LHERMITTE, F., GAUTIER, J. C., MARTEAU, R., and CHAIN, F. (1963) Troubles de la conscience et mutisme akinétique: Etude anatomo-clinique d'un ramollissement paramédian bilatéral du pédoncule cérébral et du thalamus. *Rev. Neurol. (Paris) 109:*115–131.

LICHT, S. (1949) The rehabilitation end point in hemiplegia. *Occup. Therapy and Rehab. 28:*364–367.

LINDSLEY, D. B., SCHREINER, L. H., KNOWLES, W. B., and MAGOUN, H. W. (1950) Behavioral and EEG changes following chronic brain stem lesions in the cat. *Electroenceph. Clin. Neurophysiol. 2:*483–498.

LINN, L. (1947) Sodium amytal in treatment of aphasia. *Arch. Neurol. Psychiat. 58:*357–358.

LINN, L., and STEIN, M. H. (1946) Sodium amytal in treatment of aphasia: Preliminary report. *Bull. U.S. Army Med. Dept. 5:*705–708.

LOEWENSON, RUTH (1968) "Clinical Assessment and Reliability of Clinical Ratings." Presented at the Joint Conference on Cerebrovascular Disease, Honolulu, Hawaii.

LONDON, P., and BRYAN, J. H. (1960) Theory and research on the clinical use of the Archimedes spiral. *J. Gen. Psychol. 62:*113–125.

LONGERICH, MARY C. (1955) *Helping the Aphasic To Recover His Speech: A Manual for the Family.* Los Angeles, privately printed.

LONGERICH, MARY C. (1958) *Manual for the Aphasia Patient.* New York, Macmillan.

LONGERICH, MARY C., and BORDEAUX, JEAN (1954) *Aphasia Therapeutics.* New York, Macmillan.

LORENTE DE NÓ, R. (1934) Studies on the structure of the cerebral cortex: Continuation of the study of the ammonic system. *J. Psych. Neurol. 46:*113–177.

LORENZE, E. J., and CANCRO, R. (1962) Dysfunction in visual perception with hemiplegia: Its relation to activities of daily living. *Arch. Phys. Med. 43:*514–517.

LORENZE, E. J., DEROSA, A. J., and KERNAN, E. L. (1958) Ambulation problems in hemiplegia. *Arch. Phys. Med. 39:*366–370.

LORR, M. (1961) Classification of the behavior disorders. *Ann. Rev. Psychol. 12:*195–216.

LOVETT, R. W. (1916) *The Treatment of Infantile Paralysis.* Philadelphia, Blakiston.

LOWENTHAL, M., TOBIS, J., and HOWARD, I. R. (1959) An analysis of the rehabilitation needs and prognosis of 232 cases of cerebral vascular accident. *Arch. Phys. Med. 40:*183–186.

LURIA, A. R. (1963) *Restoration of Function After Brain Injury*, trans. by Basil Haigh. New York, Macmillan.

LURIA, A. R. (1965) Two kinds of motor perseveration in massive injury to the frontal lobes. *Brain 88*:1–10.

LURIA, A. R. (1966) *Higher Cortical Functions in Man.* New York, Basic.

McDONALD, R. D., and BURNS, S. B. (1964) Visual vigilance and brain-damage: An empirical study. *J. Neurol. Neurosurg. Psychiat. 27*:206–211.

McFARLAND, J. H. (1968) "The Effect of Stimulus-Guided Eye Movements on Visual Form Recognition." Presented at meeting of Eastern Psychological Association, Philadelphia.

McFIE, J., PIERCY, M. F., and ZANGWILL, O. L. (1950) Visual-spatial agnosia associated with lesions of the right cerebral hemisphere. *Brain* 167–190.

MACLEAN, P. D., and DELGADO, J. M. R. (1953) Electrical and chemical stimulation of frontotemporal portion of limbic system in the waking animal. *Electroenceph. Clin. Neurophysiol. 5*:91–100.

MACRITCHIE, K., and ENGEL, G. L. (1968) Psychological factors in patients with cerebrovascular accident (stroke). Unpublished manuscript.

MAGOUN, H. W. (1958) *The Waking Brain.* Springfield, Ill., Thomas.

MAIER, N. R. F. (1963) "Selector-Integrator Mechanisms in Behavior," in *Principles of Animal Psychology*, ed. by Maier, N. R. F., and Schneirla, T. C. New York, Dover Books, pp. 621–649.

MARKS, M., TAYLOR, MARTHA, and RUSK, H. A. (1957) Rehabilitation of the aphasic patient: A survey of three years' experience in a rehabilitation setting. *Arch. Phys. Med. 38*:219–226.

MARSHALL, J., and SHAW, D. A. (1959) The natural history of cerebrovascular disease. *Brit. Med. J. 1*:1614–1617.

MARTIN, M. J., WHISNANT, J. P., and SAYRE, G. P. (1960) Occlusive vascular disease in the extracranial cerebral circulation. *Arch. Neurol. (Chicago) 3*:530–538.

MASLAND, R. L. (1968) "A National View of Developments in Stroke," in *Proceedings, Conference Workshop on Regional Medical Programs.* Public Health Service Publication No. 1774. Washington, D.C., G.P.O., vol. 1, pp. 59–66.

MATTHEWS, C. G., GUERTIN, W. H., and REITAN, R. M. (1962) Wechsler-Bellevue subtest mean rank orders in diverse diagnostic groups. *Psychol. Rep. 11*:3–9.

MATTHEWS, C. G., and REITAN, R. M. (1964) Correlations of Wechsler-Bellevue rank orders of subtest means in lateralized and non-lateralized brain-damaged groups. *Percept. Motor Skills, 19*:391–399.

MEDNICK, S. A. (1955) Distortions in the gradient of stimulus generalization related to cortical brain-damage and schizophrenia. *J. Abnorm. Soc. Psychol. 51*:536–542.

MEDNICK, S. A., and FREEDMAN, J. (1960) Stimulus generalization. *Psychol. Bull. 57:*169–201.

MEIER, M. J. (1967) "Readaptation to Reversal and Inversion of Visual Space in Patients with Focal Cerebral Lesions." *Proceedings, Second Pan American Congress in Neurology,* San Juan, Puerto Rico.

MEIER, M. J. (1969) "The Regional Localization Hypothesis and Personality Changes Associated with Focal Cerebral Lesions and Ablations," in *Recent Developments in the Use of the MMPI,* ed. by Butcher, J. N. New York, McGraw-Hill.

MEIER, M. J., and FRENCH, L. A. (1964a) Caudality scale changes following unilateral temporal lobectomy. *J. Clin. Psychol. 20:*464–467.

MEIER, M. J., and FRENCH, L. A. (1964b) Changes in MMPI scale scores and an index of psychopathology following unilateral temporal lobectomy for epilepsy. *Epilepsia 6:*263–273.

MEIER, M. J., and FRENCH, L. A. (1965a) Lateralized deficits in complex visual discrimination and bilateral transfer of reminiscence following unilateral temporal lobectomy. *Neuropsychologia 3:*261–272.

MEIER, M. J., and FRENCH, L. A. (1965b) Some personality correlates of unilateral and bilateral EEG abnormalities in psychomotor epileptics. *J. Clin. Psychol. 21:*3–9.

MEIER, M. J., and FRENCH, L. A. (1966a) Longitudinal assessment of intellectual functioning following unilateral temporal lobectomy. *J. Clin. Psychol. 22:*22–27.

MEIER, M. J., and FRENCH, L. A. (1966b) Readaptation to prismatic rotations of visual space as a function of lesion laterality and extratemporal EEG spike activity after temporal lobectomy. *Neuropsychologia 4:*151–157.

MEIER, M. J., and OKAYAMA, M. (1966) "Comparative Investigation of Intellectual Deficits Associated with Cerebrovascular Disease in the United States and Japan." Presented at the Midwestern Psychological Association meeting, Chicago.

MEIER, M. J., and RESCH, J. A. (1966) Readaptation to prismatic visual space rotation in predicting neurological outcome in acute cerebrovascular disease. *Proc. XVIIIth Int Cong. Psychol. 2:*165–166.

MEIER, M. J., and RESCH, J. A. (1967) Behavioral prediction of short-term neurologic change following acute onset of cerebrovascular symptoms. *Mayo Clinic Proc. 42:*641–647.

MEIER, M. J., and STORY, J. L. (1967) Selective impairment of Porteus Maze Test performance after right subthalamotomy. *Neuropsychologia 5:*181–189.

MESSIMY, R. (1953) Hallucinations in prefrontal pathology. *Presse Méd. 61:*52–54.

METTLER, F. A. (1949) *Selective Partial Ablation of the Frontal Cortex.* New York, Hoeber.

MEYER, A. (1909–1910) "The Present Status of Aphasia and Apraxia." *Harvey Lectures.* New York, Lippincott. Reprinted in *The Collected Papers of Adolf Meyer,* ed. by Winters, E. Baltimore, Johns Hopkins Press, 1950.

MEYER, J. S., and BARRON, D. W. (1960) Apraxia of gait: A clinico-physiological study. *Brain 83:*261–284.

MEYER, V. (1957) Critique of psychological approaches to brain damage. *J. Ment. Sci. 103:*80–109.

MEYER, V. (1960) "Psychological Effects of Brain Damage," in *Handbook of Abnormal Psychology,* ed. by Eysenck, H. J. New York, Basic.

MEYER, V., and JONES, H. G. (1957) Patterns of cognitive test performance as functions of the lateral localization of cerebral abnormalities in the temporal lobe. *J. Ment. Sci. 103:*758–772.

MEYER, V., and YATES, A. J. (1955) Intellectual changes following temporal lobectomy for psychomotor epilepsy; preliminary communication. *J. Neurol. Neurosurg. Psychiat. 18:*44–52.

MEYERSON, L. (1965) *Shaping Walking Behavior in a Child with Cerebral Palsy.* Film presented at workshop of directors of psychology training programs sponsored by Vocational Rehabilitation Administration, Tempe, Arizona State University, March 12.

MILLER, C. R., EYMAN, R. K., and DINGMAN, H. F. (1961) Factor analysis, latent structure analysis and mental typology. *Brit. J. Statist. Psychol. 14:*29–34.

MILLIKAN, C. H. (1967) Psychoneurologic research needs in evaluation of patients with cerebrovascular accidents. *Mayo Clin. Proc. 42:*637–647.

MILNER, BRENDA (1954) Intellectual functions of the temporal lobes. *Psychol. Bull. 51:*42–62.

MILNER, BRENDA (1958) Psychological defects produced by temporal-lobe excision. *Res. Publ. Ass. Res. Nerv. Ment. Dis. 36:*244–257.

MILNER, BRENDA (1962) "Laterality Effects in Audition," in *Interhemispheric Relations and Cerebral Dominance,* ed. by Mountcastle, V. B. Baltimore, Johns Hopkins Press, pp. 177–195.

MILNER, BRENDA (1964) "Some Effects of Frontal Lobectomy in Man," in *The Frontal Granular Cortex and Behavior,* ed. by Warren, J. M., and Akert, K. New York, McGraw-Hill, pp. 313–334.

MILNER, BRENDA (1965) Visually-guided maze learning in man: Effects of bilateral hippocampal, bilateral frontal, and unilateral cerebral lesions. *Neuropsychologia 3:*317–338.

MILNER, BRENDA (1967) "Brain Mechanisms Suggested by the Studies of the Temporal Lobes," in *Brain Mechanisms Underlying Speech and Language,* ed. by Darley, F. L. New York, Grune.

MILNER, BRENDA, and KIMURA, DOREEN (1964) "Dissociable Verbal Learning Deficits After Unilateral Temporal Lobectomy in Man." Paper read at Eastern Psychological Association Meeting, Philadelphia.

MILNER, BRENDA, TAYLOR, L., and CORKIN, SUZANNE (1967) "Tactual Pattern Recognition After Differential Unilateral Cortical Excisions." Paper presented at the Eastern Psychological Association Meeting, Boston.

MISHKIN, M., and PRIBRAM, K. H. (1954) Visual discrimination performance following partial ablations of the temporal lobe. I. Ventral vs. lateral. *J. Comp. Physiol. Psychol. 47:*14–20.

MOFFETT, A., ETTLINGER, G., MORTON, H. B., and PIERCY, M. F. (1967) Tactile discrimination performance in the monkey: The effect of ablation of various subdivisions of posterior parietal cortex. *Cortex 3:*59–96.

MOORE, P., and SCHUELL, HILDRED (n.d.) *The Language Master—Handbook for Aphasia.* Language Stimulation Series. New York, McGraw-Hill.

MORISON, R. S., and DEMPSEY, E. W. (1942) A study of thalamo-cortical relations. *Amer. J. Physiol. 135:*281–292.

MORUZZI, G., and MAGOUN, H. W. (1949) Brain stem reticular formation and activation of the EEG. *Electroenceph. Clin. Neurophysiol. 1:*455–473.

MOSKOWITZ, E., BISHOP, H. F., PE, H., and SHIBUTANI, K. (1958) Posthemiplegic reflex sympathetic dystrophy. *J. Amer. Med. Ass. 167:*836–838.

MOSKOWITZ, E., and PORTER, J. I. (1963) Peripheral nerve lesions in the upper extremity in hemiplegic patients. *New Eng. J. Med. 269:*776–778.

MOUNTCASTLE, V. B. (1962) *Interhemispheric Relations and Cerebral Dominance.* Baltimore, Johns Hopkins Press.

NAUTA, W. J. H. (1953) Some projections of the medial wall of the hemisphere in the rat's brain (cortical areas 32 and 25, 24 and 29). *Anat. Rec. 115:*352.

NAUTA, W. J. H. (1956) An experimental study of the fornix system in the rat. *J. Comp. Neurol. 104:*247–271.

NAUTA, W. J. H., and WHITLOCK, D. G. (1954) "An Anatomical Analysis of the Non-Specific Thalamic Projection System," in *Brain Mechanism and Consciousness: A Symposium.* Council for International Organizations of Medical Science. Oxford, Blackwell, pp. 81–116.

NIELSEN, J. M., and JACOBS, L. L. (1951) Bilateral lesions of the anterior cingulate gyri: Report of case. *Bull. Los Angeles Neurol. Soc. 16:*231–234.

NOBLE, C. E. (1968) The learning of psychomotor skills. *Ann. Rev. Psychol. 19:*203–250.

NODINE, J. H., SHULKIN, M. W., SLAP, J. W., LEVINE, M., and FREIBERG, K. (1967) Double-blind study of effect of ribonucleic acid in senile brain disease. *Amer. J. Psychiat. 123:*1257–1259.

NOYES, A. P., and KOLB, L. C. (1968) *Modern Clinical Psychiatry,* 6th ed. Philadelphia, Saunders, pp. 221–222.

OLDS, J. (1958) "Adaptive Functions of Paleocortical and Related Structures," in *Biological and Biochemical Bases of Behavior,* ed. by Harlow, H. F., and Woolsey, C. N. Madison, University of Wisconsin Press, pp. 237–262.

PAGE, I. H. (1968) What about strokes? *Modern Medicine,* July, pp. 45–46.

PANZA, J. M. (1966) "Factors Accounting for Successful Vocational Placement of Persons with Stroke," in *Research Needs in Rehabilitation of Patients with Stroke,* ed. by Fields, W. S., and Spencer, W. A. Houston, Texas Medical Center.

PATERSON, A., and ZANGWILL, O. L. (1944) Disorders of visual space perception associated with lesions of the right cerebral hemisphere. *Brain 67:*331–358.

PEARCE, J. M., GUBBAY, S. S., and WALTON, J. N. (1965) Long-term anticoagulant therapy in transient cerebral ischaemic attacks. *Lancet 1:*6–9.

PENFIELD, W., and ROBERTS, L. (1959) *Speech and Brain Mechanisms.* Princeton, Princeton University Press.

PERCHERON, G. M. J. (1966) "Etude anatomique de thalamus de l'homme adulte et de sa vascularisation artérielle." Thesis, Paris.

PESZCZYNSKI, M., and BRUELL, J. (1960) Measuring disability in patients with hemiplegia. *Geriatrics 15:*750–757.

PETERSON, JEAN C., and OLSEN, ANN P. (1964) *Language Problems after a Stroke.* Minneapolis, Kenny Rehabilitation Institute.

PIERCY, M. (1964) The effects of cerebral lesions on intellectual function: A review of current research trends. *Brit. J. Psychiat. 110:*310–352.

PIERCY, M., and SMYTH, V. O. (1962) Right hemisphere dominance for certain nonverbal intellectual tasks. *Brain 85:*775–790.

PLUM, F., and POSNER, J. B. (1966) *The Diagnosis of Stupor and Coma.* Philadelphia, Davis.

POPPELREUTER, W. (1917) *Die psychischen Schädigungen durch Kopfschuss im Kriege* 1914. Band I. *Die Störungen der niederen und höheren Sehleistungen durch Verletzungen des Occipitalhirns.* Leipzig, Voss.

POPPEN, J. L. (1939) Ligation of the left anterior cerebral artery: Its hazards and means of avoidance of its complications. *Arch. Neurol. Psychiat. 41:*495–503.

PORCH, B. E. (1967) *Porch Index of Communicative Ability.* Palo Alto, Consulting Psychologists Press.

PORTEUS, S. D. (1933) *The Maze Test and Mental Differences.* Vineland, Smith Printing and Publishing House.

PORTEUS, S. D. (1955) *The Maze Test: Recent Advances.* Palo Alto, Pacific Books.

PORTEUS, S. D. (1959) *The Maze Test and Clinical Psychology.* Palo Alto, Pacific Books.

Poser, C. M., Zosa, A. M., Gomez, A. J., and Hardin, C. A. (1964) Cervicocephalic angiography for cerebrovascular insufficiency. *Acta Neurol. Scand. 40*:321–336.

Rae, J. W., Smith, E. M., and Lenzce, A. (1962) Results of a rehabilitation program for geriatric patients in county hospitals. *J. Amer. Med. Ass. 180*:463–466.

Ragoff, J. B., Cooney, D. V., and Kutner, B. (1964) Hemiplegia: A study of home rehabilitation. *J. Chronic Dis. 17*:539–550.

Ramón y Cajal, S. (1909) *Histologie du Système Nerveux de L'homme et des Vertébrés.* Paris, Maloine.

Rankin, J. (1957) Cerebral vascular accidents in patients over the age of 60: General considerations. *Scot. Med. J. 2*:127–136.

Raven, J. C. (1958) *Guide to Using the Coloured Progressive Matrices.* London, Lewis.

Reitan, R. M. (1955a) Certain differential effects of left and right cerebral lesions in human adults. *J. Comp. Physiol. Psychol. 48*:474–477.

Reitan, R. M. (1955b) Investigation of the validity of Halstead's measures of biological intelligence. *Arch. Neurol. Psychiat. 73*:28–35.

Reitan, R. M. (1958a) Qualitative versus quantitative mental changes following brain damage. *J. Psychol. 46*:339–346.

Reitan, R. M. (1958b) Validity of the trail making test as an indicator of organic brain damage. *Percept. Motor Skills 8*:271–276.

Reitan, R. M. (1962) Psychological deficit. *Ann. Rev. Psychol. 13*:415–444.

Reitan, R. M. (1964) "Psychological Deficits Resulting From Cerebral Lesions in Man," in *The Frontal Granular Cortex and Behavior,* ed. by Warren, J. M., and Akert, K. New York, McGraw-Hill, pp. 295–312.

Reitan, R. M., and Tarshes, E. L. (1959) Differential effects of lateralized brain lesions on the trail making test. *J. Nerv. Ment. Dis. 129*:257–262.

Riese, W. (1948) Aphasia in brain tumors. *Confin. Neurol. 9*:64–79.

Riklan, M., and Levita, E. (1965) Laterality of subcortical involvement and psychological functions. *Psychol. Bull. 64*:217–224.

Riklan, M., Levita, E., and Diller, L. (1961) Psychologic studies in neurologic disease—review: Parkinson's disease and multiple sclerosis. *J. Amer. Geriat. Soc. 9*:857–867.

Riklan, M., Weiner, J., and Diller, L. (1959) Somato-psychologic studies in Parkinson's disease. I. An investigation into the relationship of certain disease factors to psychological functions. *J. Nerv. Ment. Dis. 129*:263–272.

Rodda, R., and Denny-Brown, D. (1966) Cerebral arterioles in experimental hypertension. II. Development of arteriolonecrosis. *Amer. J. Path. 49*:365–381.

Rood, M. (1962) "The Use of Sensory Receptors to Activate, Facilitate and Inhibit Motor Response Autonomic and Somatic in Developmental Sequence," in *Approaches to Treatment of Patients with Neuromuscular Dysfunction,* ed. by Sattley, C. Dubuque, Iowa, W. C. Brown, pp. 26–37.

Rosenberg, B. (1965) The performance of aphasics on automated visuo-perceptual discrimination, training, and transfer tasks. *J. Speech Hearing Res. 8:*165–181.

Rosenblatt, H. A. (1961) Rehabilitation of the hemiplegic patient. *Penn. Med. J. 64:*56–60.

Rosenthal, A. M., Pearson, L., Medenica, B., Manaster, A., and Smith, C. S. (1965) Correlation of perceptual factors with rehabilitation of hemiplegic patients. *Arch. Phys. Med. 46:*461–466.

Rosvold, H. E., Mirsky, A. F., Sarason, I., Bransome, E. D., Jr., and Beck, L. H. (1956) A continuous performance test for brain damage. *J. Consult. Psych. 20:*343–350.

Rothschild, D. (1956) "Senile Psychoses and Psychoses with Cerebral Arteriosclerosis," in *Mental Disorders in Later Life,* 2nd ed., ed. by Kaplan, O. J. Stanford, Stanford University Press, pp. 289–331.

Ruch, T. C. (1961) "Neurophysiology of Emotion and Motivation," in *Neurophysiology,* ed. by Ruch, T. C., Patton, H. D., Woodbury, J. W. and Towe, A. L. Philadelphia, Saunders, pp. 483–499.

Rusk, H. A. (1964) *Rehabilitation Medicine.* St. Louis, Mosby.

Saetveit, J. G., Lewis, D., and Seashore, C. E. (1940) *Revision of the Seashore Measure of Musical Talents.* University of Iowa Studies No. 65. Iowa City, University of Iowa Press.

Sands, Elaine, Sarno, Martha T., and Shankweiler, D. (1969) Long-term assessment of language function in aphasia due to stroke. *Arch. Phys. Med. 50:*202–206.

Sarno, M. T. (1964) Language Therapy in *The Aphasic Adult: Evaluation and Rehabilitation* ed. by Burr, H. G. Charlottesville, Va., Wayside Press.

Sarno, Martha T., and Sands, Elaine (1967) A new approach to the study and treatment of the aphasic patient with severe verbal impairment. *Arch. Phys. Med. 48:*689.

Satz, P. (1966a) A block rotation task: The application of multivariate and decision theory analysis for the prediction of organic brain disorder. *Psychol. Monogr. 80:*1–29.

Satz, P. (1966b) Specific and nonspecific effects of brain lesions in man. *J. Abnorm. Psych. 71:*61–70.

Scargill, M. H. (1954) Modern linguistics and recovery from aphasia. *J. Speech Hearing Dis. 19:*507–513.

Schmale, A. H., Jr., and Engel, G. L. (1967) The giving up—given up complex illustrated on film. *Arch. Gen. Psychiat. 17:*135–145.

SCHOENING, H. A. (1965) *The Kenny Self-Care Evaluation: A Numerical Measure of Independence in Activities of Daily Living.* Minneapolis, American Rehabilitation Foundation.

SCHOENING, H. A., ANDEREGG, L., BERGSTROM, D., FONDA, M., STEINKE, N., and ULRICH, P. (1965) Numerical scoring of self-care status of patients. *Arch. Phys. Med. 46*:689–697.

SCHOENING, H. A., and IVERSON, I. A. (1968) Numerical scoring of self-care status: A study of the Kenny self-care evaluation. *Arch. Phys. Med. 49*:221–229.

SCHUBERT, J. (1967) Effect of training on the performance of the WISC "Block Design" test. *Brit. J. Soc. Clin. Psychol. 6*:144–149.

SCHUELL, HILDRED (1965) *Minnesota Test for Differential Diagnosis of Aphasia.* Minneapolis, University of Minnesota Press.

SCHUELL, HILDRED, and JENKINS, J. J. (1959) The nature of language deficit in aphasia. *Psych. Rev. 66*:45–67.

SCHUELL, HILDRED, JENKINS, J. J., and CARROLL, J. B. (1961) A factor analysis of the Minnesota test for differential diagnosis of aphasia. *J. Speech Hearing Res. 4*:30–36.

SCHUELL, HILDRED, JENKINS, J. J., and JIMÉNEZ-PABON, E. (1964) *Aphasia in Adults.* New York, Hoeber.

SCULL, E., KOMISAR, D., LEONHARDT, H. L., and WEITZ, A. S. (1962) A follow-up study of patients discharged from a community rehabilitation center. *J. Chronic Dis. 15*:207–213.

SEMMES, J., WEINSTEIN, A. S., GHENT, L., and TEUBER, H. L. (1960) *Somatosensory Changes after Penetrating Wounds in Man.* Cambridge, Mass., Harvard University Press.

SHANKWEILER, D. P. (1959) Effects of success and failure instructions on reaction time in patients with brain damage. *J. Comp. Physiol. Psychol. 52*:546–549.

SHANKWEILER, D. (1966) Effects of temporal-lobe damage on perception of dichotically presented melodies. *J. Comp. Physiol. Psychol. 62*:115–119

SHANKWEILER, D. P., and HARRIS, K. S. (1966) An experimental approach to the problem of articulation in aphasia. *Cortex 2*:277–292.

SHANKWEILER, D. P., HARRIS, K. S., and TAYLOR, M. L. (1968) Electromyographic studies of articulation in aphasia. *Arch. Phys. Med. 49*:1–8.

SHAPIRO, M. B. (1951) Experimental studies of a perceptual anomaly. I. Initial experiments. *J. Ment. Sci. 97*:90–110.

SHAPIRO, M. B. (1952) Experimental studies of a perceptual anomaly. II. Confirmatory and explanatory experiments. *J. Ment. Sci. 98*:605–617.

SHAPIRO, M. B. (1953) Experimental studies of a perceptual anomaly. III. The testing of an explanatory theory. *J. Ment. Sci. 99*:394–409.

SHEEHAN, VIVIAN M. (1946) Rehabilitation of aphasics in an army hospital. *J. Speech Dis. 11*:149–157.

SHEER, D. E. (1956) *Studies in Topectomy.* New York, Grune.

Shuttleworth, E. C., and Morris, C. E. (1966) The transient global amnesia syndrome: A defect in the second stage of memory in man. *Arch. Neurol. (Chicago) 15:*515–520.

Silverstein, A., and Hollin, S. (1965) Internal carotid vs. middle cerebral artery occlusions. *Arch. Neurol. (Chicago) 12:*468–471.

Skinner, B. F. (1954) The science of learning and the art of teaching. *Harvard Educ. Rev. 24:*86–97.

Skinner, B. F. (1957) *Verbal Behavior.* New York, Appleton.

Skinner, B. F. (1958) Teaching machines. *Science 128:*969–977.

Skinner, B. F. (1961) Why we need teaching machines. *Harvard Educ. Rev. 31:*177–398.

Skultety, F. M. (1962) Experimental mutism in dogs. *Arch. Neurol. (Chicago) 6:*235–241.

Skultety, F. M. (1965) Mutism in cats with rostral midbrain lesions. *Arch. Neurol. (Chicago) 12:*211–225.

Skultety, F. M. (1968) Clinical and experimental aspects of akinetic mutism. *Arch. Neurol. (Chicago) 19:*1–14.

Smith, A. (1960) Changes in Porteus Maze scores of brain-operated schizophrenics after an eight-year interval. *J. Ment. Sci. 106:*967–978.

Smith, A. (1965) Verbal and nonverbal test performances of patients with "acute" lateralized brain lesions (tumors). *J. Nerv. Ment. Dis. 141:*517–523.

Smith, A. (1966) Certain hypothesized hemispheric differences in language and visual functions in human adults. *Cortex 2:*109–126.

Smith, K. U., and Smith, W. M. (1962) *Perception and Motion: An Analysis of Space-Structured Behavior.* Philadelphia, Saunders.

Smith, K. U., and Wehrkamp, R. (1951) Universal motion analyzer applied to psychomotor performance. *Science 113:*242–246.

Smith, S., and Turton, E. C. (1951) Restoration of speech in severe aphasia by intravenous and oral priscol. *Brit. Med. J. 2:*891–892.

Spellacy, F. J. (1969) "Ear Preference in the Dichotic Presentation of Patterned Nonverbal Stimuli." Ph.D. Dissertation, University of Victoria.

Spieth, W. (1962) Abnormally slow perceptual-motor task performances in individuals with stable, mild to moderate heart disease. *Aerospace Med. 33:*370.

Spieth, W. (1967) Reaction to cardiovascular change. *Mayo Clinic Proc. 42:*632–636.

Spreen, O., and Benton, A. L. (1968a) Neurosensory Center Comprehensive Examination for Aphasia. University of Victoria, B.C., Canada.

Spreen, O., and Benton, A. L. (1968b) A factorial analysis of aphasic test performance. Unpublished study.

Spreen, O., Benton, A. L., and Van Allen, M. W. (1966) Dissociation of visual and tactile naming in amnesic aphasia. *Neurology (Minneap.) 16:*807–814.

STEPHENSON, W. (1953) *The Study of Behavior, Q-technique and its Methodology,* Chicago, University of Chicago Press.

STERN, P. H., McDOWELL, F., MILLER, J. M., and ELKIN, R. D. (1969) "Quantitative Testing of Motility Defects of Patients with Stroke." *Arch. Phys. Med. 50:*320–325.

STOICHEFF, MARGARET L. (1960) Motivating instructions and language performance of dysphasic subjects. *J. Speech Hearing Res. 3:*75–85.

SZAFRAN, J. (1963) Age differences in choice reaction time and cardio-vascular status among pilots. *Nature 200:*904–906.

SZAFRAN, J. (1965) Age differences in the rate of gain of information, signal-detection strategy, and cardiovascular status among pilots. *Amer. Psychol. 20:*581.

TALLAND, G. A., HAGEN, D. Q., and JAMES, M. (1967) Performance tests of amnesic patients with cylert. *J. Nerv. Ment. Dis. 144:*421–429.

TAYLOR, MARTHA L. (1958) *Understanding Aphasia.* New York, Institute of Physical Medicine and Rehabilitation.

TAYLOR, MARTHA L. (1964) "Language Therapy," in *The Aphasic Adult: Evaluation and Rehabilitation,* ed. by Burr, Helen G. Charlottesville, Va., Wayside Press.

TAYLOR, MARTHA L. (1965) A measurement of functional communication in aphasia. *Arch. Phys. Med. 46:*101–107.

TAYLOR, MARTHA L., and MARKS, M. D. (1959) *Aphasia Rehabilitation Manual and Therapy Kit,* 2nd ed. New York, Saxon Press.

TELLEGEN, A., and BRIGGS, P. F. (1967) Old wine in new skins: Grouping Wechsler subtests into new scales. *J. Consult. Psychol. 31:*499–506.

TERZIAN, H., and DALLE ORE, G. (1955) Syndrome of Klüver and Bucy: Reproduced in man by bilateral removal of the temporal lobes. *Neurology (Minneap.) 5:*373–380.

TEUBER, H.-L. (1955) Physiological psychology. *Ann. Rev. Psychol. 6:*267–296.

TEUBER, H.-L. (1959) "Some Alterations in Behavior After Cerebral Lesions in Man," in *Evolution of Nervous Control from Primitive Organisms to Man,* ed. by Bass, A. D. American Association for the Advancement of Science, Washington, D.C.

TEUBER, H.-L. (1960) "Perception," in *Handbook of Physiology, Sect. I, Neurophysiology,* Baltimore, Williams & Wilkins, vol. 3, pp. 1595–1668.

TEUBER, H.-L. (1962) "Effects of Brain Wounds Implicating Right or Left Hemisphere in Man," in *Interhemispheric Relations and Cerebral Dominance,* ed. by Mountcastle, V. B. Baltimore, Johns Hopkins Press, pp. 131–157.

TEUBER, H.-L. (1964) "The Riddle of Frontal Lobe Function in Man," in *The Frontal Granular Cortex and Behavior,* ed. by Warren, J. M., and Akert, K. New York, McGraw-Hill, pp. 410–444.

TEUBER, H.-L., BATTERSBY, W. S., and BENDER, M. B. (1949). Changes in visual searching performance following cerebral lesions. *Amer. J. Physiol. 159:*592–603.

TEUBER, H.-L., BATTERSBY, W. S., and BENDER, M. B. (1951) Performance of complex visual tasks after cerebral lesions. *J. Nerv. Ment. Dis. 114:*413–429.

TEUBER, H.-L., and MISHKIN, M. (1954) Judgment of visual and postural vertical after brain injury. *J. Psychol. 38:*161–175.

THOMAS, C. W., SPANGLER, D. P., and IZUTSU, S. (1961) Some fundamental proportions in the construction of evaluation units in vocational rehabilitation, *Personn. Guid. J. 39:*586–590.

THOMPSON, G. N. (1951) Cerebral area essential to consciousness. *Bull. Los Angeles Neurol. Soc. 16:*311–334.

TIKOFSKY, R. S., and REYNOLDS, G. L. (1962) Preliminary study: Nonverbal learning and aphasia. *J. Speech Hearing Res. 5:*133–143.

TIKOFSKY, R. S., and REYNOLDS, G. L. (1963) Further studies of nonverbal learning and aphasia. *J. Speech Hearing Res. 6:*329–337.

TOOLE, J. F., and PATEL, A. M. (1967) *Cerebrovascular Disorders.* New York, McGraw-Hill.

TOURTELLOTTE, W. W., HAERER, A. F., SIMPSON, J. F., KUZMA, J. W., and SIKORSKI, J. (1965) Quantitative clinical neurological testing. I. A study of a battery of tests designed to evaluate in part the neurological function of patients with multiple sclerosis and its use in a therapeutic trial. *Ann. N.Y. Acad. Sci. 122:*480–505.

TREANOR, W., and PSAKI, R. (1954) Patterns of restitution of motor functions. *Phys. Ther. Rev. 34:*610–617.

TWITCHELL, T. E. (1951) The restoration of motor function following hemiplegia in man. *Brain 74:*443–480.

ULLMAN, M. (1961) Reactive states following strokes. *J. Arkansas Med. Soc. 58:*265–270.

ULLMAN, M. (1962) *Behavioral Changes in Patients Following Strokes.* Springfield, Ill., Thomas.

ULLMAN, M., and GRUEN, A. (1961) Behavioral changes in patients with strokes. *Amer. J. Psychiat. 117:*1004–1009.

VAN ALLEN, M. W., BENTON, A. L., and GORDON, MUSETTA, C. (1966) Temporal discrimination in brain-damaged patients. *Neuropsychologia 4:*159–167.

VAN BUSKIRK, C. (1954) Return of motor function in hemiplegia. *Neurology (Minneap.) 4:*919–928.

VAN BUSKIRK, C., and WEBSTER, D. (1955) Prognostic value of sensory defect in rehabilitation of hemiplegics. *Neurology (Minneap.) 5:*407–411.

VANDER EECKEN, H. M., and ADAMS, R. D. (1953) Anatomy and functional significance of the meningeal arterial anastomoses of human brain. *J. Neuropath. Exp. Neurol. 12:*132–157.

VAUGHN, H. G. J., and COSTA, L. D. (1962) Performance of patients with lateralized cerebral lesions. II. Sensory and motor tests. *J. Nerv. Ment. Dis. 134:*237–244.

VICTOR, M., ANGEVINE, J. B., MANCALL, E. L., and FISHER, C. M. (1961) Memory loss with lesions of hippocampal formation. *Arch. Neurol. (Chicago) 5:*244–263.

VIGNOLO, L. A. (1965) Evolution of aphasia and language rehabilitation: A retrospective exploratory study. *Cortex 1:*344–367.

VON BÉKÉSY, G. (1967) *Sensory Inhibition.* Princeton, Princeton Univ. Press.

VON MONAKOW, C. (1911) Lokalisation der Hirnfunktionen. *J. Neurol. Psychiat. 17:*185–200.

VON MONAKOW, C. (1914) *Die Lokalisation im Grosshirn und der Abbau der Funktion durch Kortikale Herde.* Wiesbaden, Bergmann.

WACHTEL, P. (1967) Conceptions of broad and narrow attention. *Psychol. Bull. 68:*417–430.

WARRINGTON, E. K. (1962) The completion of visual forms across hemianopic field defects. *J. Neurol. Neurosurg. Psychiat. 25:*208–217.

WARRINGTON, E. K., and JAMES, M. (1967) An experimental investigation of facial recognition in patients with unilateral cerebral lesions. *Cortex 3:*317–326.

WECHSLER, D. (1955) *Manual for the Wechsler Adult Intelligence Scale.* New York, The Psychological Corporation.

WEINSTEIN, E. A., and COLE, M. (1963) "Concepts of Anosognosia," in *Problems of Dynamic Neurology,* ed. by Halpern, L. Jerusalem, Hebrew University Hadassah Medical School, pp. 254–273.

WEINSTEIN, E. A., and KAHN, R. L. (1950) Syndrome of anosognosia. *Arch. Neurol. Psychiat. 64:*772–791.

WEINSTEIN, E. A., and KAHN, R. L. (1955) *Denial of Illness,* Springfield, Ill., Thomas.

WEINSTEIN, E. A., KAHN, R. L., MALITZ, S., and ROSANSKI, J. (1954) Delusional reduplication of parts of the body. *Brain 77:*45–60.

WEINSTEIN, S. (1962) "Differences in Effects of Brain Wounds Implicating Right or Left Hemispheres: Differential Effects of Certain Intellectual and Complex Perceptual Functions," in *Interhemispheric Relations and Cerebral Dominance,* ed. by Mountcastle, V. B. Baltimore, Johns Hopkins Press, pp. 159–176.

WEISS, J. M., CHATHAM, L. R., and SCHAIE, K. W. (1961) Symptom formation associated with aging: Dynamic pattern. *Arch. Gen. Psychiat. 4:*22–29.

WELCH, K., and STUTEVILLE, P. (1958) Experimental production of unilateral neglect in monkeys. *Brain 81:*341–347.

WELFORD, A. T. (1959) "Psychomotor Performance," in *Handbook of Ageing and the Individual,* ed. by Birren, J. E. Chicago, University of Chicago Press, pp. 562–613.

WELFORD, A. T., and BIRREN, J. (1965) *Behavior, Ageing and the Nervous System,* Springfield, Ill., Thomas.

WELLS, F. L., and RUESCH, J. (1945) *Mental Examiner's Handbook.* New York, The Psychological Corporation.

WEPMAN, J. M. (1947) The organization of therapy for aphasia; inpatient treatment center. *J. Speech Hearing Dis. 12:*405–409.

WEPMAN, J. M. (1951) *Recovery from Aphasia.* New York, Ronald Press Co.

WEPMAN, J. M. (1953) A conceptual model for the processes involved in recovery from aphasia. *J. Speech Hearing Dis. 18:*4–13.

WEPMAN, J. M., and JONES, L. V. (1961) *Studies in Aphasia: An Approach to Testing.* Chicago, Education-Industry Series.

WEPMAN, J. M., and VAN PELT, DORIS (1955) A theory of cerebral language disorders based on therapy. *Folia Phoniatrica 7:*223–235.

WERNER, H., and WEIR, A. (1956) The figure-ground syndrome in the brain-injured child. *Int. Rec. Med. 169:*363–367.

WERNICKE, C. (1874) *Der aphasische Symptomencomplex.* Breslau, Max Cohn und Weigert.

WESTCOTT, E. J. (1967) Traditional exercise regimens for the hemiplegic patient. *Amer. J. Phys. Med. 46:*1012–1023.

WHEELER, L., BURKE, C. J., and REITAN, R. M. (1963) An application of discriminant functions to the problem of predicting brain damage using behavioral variables. *Percept. Motor Skills Monogr.* (Suppl.) *16:*417–440.

WHEELER, L., and REITAN, R. M. (1963) Discriminant functions applied to the problem of predicting cerebral damage from behavioral tests: A cross-validation study. *Percept. Motor Skills Monogr.* (Suppl.) *16:*681–701.

WICKES, I. G. (1958) Treatment of persistent eneuresis with the electric buzzer. *Arch. Dis. Child. 33:*160–164.

WILLETT, R. A. (1961) "The Effects of Psychosurgical Procedures on Behavior," in *Handbook of Abnormal Psychology,* ed. by Eysenck, H. J. New York, Basic, pp. 566–610.

WILLIAMS, H., GIESEKING, C., and LUBIN, A. (1961) Interaction of brain injury with peripheral vision and set. *J. Consult. Psychol. 25:*543–548.

WILLIAMS, H., LUBIN, A., GIESEKING, C., and RUBENSTEIN, I. (1956) The relations of brain injury and visual perception to block design rotation. *J. Consult. Psychol 20:*275–280.

WILLIAMS, N. (1967) Correlation between copying ability and dressing activities in hemiplegia. *Amer. J. Phys. Med. 46:*1332–1338.

Wilson, W. P., and Hohman, L. B. (1953) Intravenous sodium iodide in treatment of advanced senile psychosis and arteriosclerotic cerebrovascular disease. *J. Nerv. Ment. Dis. 118:*351–354.

Wolff, H. G. (1961) Man's nervous system and disease. *Arch. Neurol.* (*Chicago*) *5:*235–243.

Woodburne, L. S. (1967) Partial analysis of the neural elements in posture and locomotion. *Psych. Bull. 68:*121–148.

Wyke, M., and Ettlinger, G. (1961) Efficiency of recognition in left and right visual fields. *Arch. Neurol.* (*Chicago*) *5:*659–665.

Wylie, C. M. (1966) Rehabilitative care of stroke patients. *J. Amer. Med. Ass. 196:*1117–1120.

Yakovlev, P. I. (1954) Paraplegia in flexion of cerebral origin. *J. Neuropath. Exp. Neurol. 13:*267–296.

Yakovlev, P. (1968) Personal communication.

Yates, A. J. (1956) The rotation of drawings by brain-damaged patients. *J. Abnorm. Soc. Psychol. 53:*178–182.

Yates, A. J. (1966) Psychological deficit. *Ann. Rev. Psychol. 17:*111–144.

Zane, M. D. (1966) Psychiatric problems in acute stroke. *New York J. Med. 66:*2001–2004.

Zane, M. D. (1967) Changing motor performance and personality in therapeutic settings. *Bull. N.Y. Acad. Med. 43:*232–240.

Zane, M. D., and Goldman, H. (1966) Can response to double simultaneous stimulation be improved in hemiplegic patients? *J. Nerv. Ment. Dis. 142:*445–452.

Zarling, V. R. (1954) Rehabilitation in chronic neurologic disease. *Neurology* (*Minneap.*) *4:*147–156.

INDEX

71 72 73 10 9 8 7 6 5 4 3 2 1